Neck Injuries

Presented to Dr Shabbeer Qureshi,
my colleague at the GMC, with
best wishes

Springer

London
Berlin
Heidelberg
New York
Barcelona
Hong Kong
Milan
Paris
Santa Clara
Singapore
Tokyo

S.M.A. Babar

Neck Injuries

With 107 illustrations

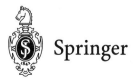

Springer

Syed Maqbool Ahmad Babar, MBBS, D Av Med (Eng), FRCS, FICA
Consultant General and Vascular Surgeon, London

ISBN 1-85233-637-4 Springer-Verlag London Berlin Heidelberg

British Library Cataloguing in Publication Data
Babar, Syed Maqbool Ahmad
    Neck injuries
    1. Neck – Wounds and injuries
    I. Title
    617.5'3'044
    ISBN 1852336374
Library of Congress Cataloging-in-Publication Data
Babar, Syed Maqbool Ahmad, 1943–
    Neck injuries/Syed Maqbool Ahmad Babar.
        p.   cm.
    Includes bibliographical references and index.
    ISBN 1-85233-637-4 (alk. paper)
    1. Neck – Wounds and injuries.   I. Title.
    [DNLM: 1. Neck Injuries. WE 708 B112n 1999]
    RD531.B23   1999
    617.5'3044–dc21
    DNLM/DLC
    for Library of Congress   99-33583

© Springer-Verlag London Limited 2000
Printed in Great Britain

The use of registered names, trademarks etc. in this publication does not imply, even in the absence of a specific statement, that such names are exempt from the relevant laws and regulations and therefore free for general use.

Product liability: The publisher can give no guarantee for information about drug dosage and application thereof contined in this book. In every individual case the respective user must check its accuracy by consulting other pharmaceutical literature.

Typesetting: Gray Publishing, Tunbridge Wells, Kent
Printed and bound at the Cromwell Press, Trowbridge, UK
34/3830-543210 Printed on acid-free paper SPIN 10733100

Dedication

This book is dedicated to my daughters, Humera and Natasha

Preface

When I started delivering lectures to the surgical postgraduates on the subject of vascular injuries of the neck, one thing led to another and very quickly I realised that there was a large gap in the understanding of an average postgraduate about various inter-related matters in this difficult subject. Here I have tried to compile such inter-related problems into a composite group, for an easy reference and a broad overview of this subject. The integrated information is designed to be principally of use to a general surgical trainee.

In the first instance, neck injuries are generally treated by trainee general surgeons and often the patient's condition does not allow for specialty co-ordination. Hence the need for the typical general surgical trainee to be conversant with the principles of management of various structures in the neck.

The book presents an easy format for quick reference and the text is supplemented with hand-drawn diagrams in relevant context. Such diagrams can be easily reproduced during surgical examinations. For a more in-depth understanding of the individual problem, the reader is advised to refer to specialist textbooks.

This book has two basic objectives. First, to comprehensively familiarise the reader with regional pathology and clinical facts relating to a seemingly simple neck injury. Second, to enable the reader to analyse the clinical problems of the patient as a whole, on the basis of factual objective findings and clinical suspicion.

I would like to thank Professor Leslie Findley, Consultant Neurologist, for giving valuable and constructive advice and encouragement.

The contents of this book should be matched with your own clinical findings. There are so few comprehensive books available on this subject that it has become necessary for me to resort to generalisation and to the use of whatever supportive literature I could gather. If you think that this book can benefit from your own experiences, I would appreciate your comments.

SMA Babar
22 Harley Street
London W1

Foreword

Complex neck injuries have always fascinated me. There is a great mystery about this subject and with so many specialties being involved in this region, the subject matter either becomes highly specialised and difficult to understand clinically or the management of the patient becomes the confusing responsibility of a variety of clinicians, which does not always do justice to the welfare of the patient.

It is refreshing, therefore, to see a comprehensive book on neck injuries, which is easy to understand from the point of view of surgical trainees, and which contains simple anatomical and surgical diagrams which are easy to follow and which can be reproduced by an examination candidate. The book covers large representative areas in the fields of general, vascular, ENT, orthopaedic, trauma, maxillofacial and neurosurgery. I found the specialty integration to be excellent.

I am particularly impressed with the layout which is easy to scan and which can lead the reader to a specific area of interest without having to go through a lot of unnecessary material. This will be of particular use to the surgical trainee seeking materials of interest in a short space of time.

This book can be used both as an aid to revision for an examination as well as a bench book on neck injuries, helping the front-line clinician involved with the primary management of neck injuries. It is not a substitute for comprehensive textbooks, which should be consulted in relevant context, but can enlighten a trainee of one specialty about the inter-related problems of an adjoining specialty.

Anthony N Mitra, MB, ChB
FRCS (Ed) General Surgery
FRCS (Eng) Otolaryngology
Consultant ENT Surgeon to
Barking, Havering and
Brentwood Group of Hospitals

Contents

1 Introduction

The first documented medical description in the available literature of a penetrating injury of the neck comes from the discovery and translation of a 5000-year-old Egyptian papyrus.[1] In this, Imhotep (the greatest of ancient Egypt's physician-cum-architects who also designed and built the step pyramid of Saqqara), vividly described a knife-inflicted oesophageal perforation, which resulted in a demonstrable mucocutaneous fistula.

In the modern era of high-speed transportation, sophisticated weaponry and increasing incidence of criminal violence, neck injuries have assumed a major role in the sphere of traumatology.

Neck injury does not usually occur in isolation, but its presence may dictate the plan of overall management. Some neck injuries are instantaneously fatal because of the anatomical vulnerability of the neck and because of the delicate nature of the unprotected viscera either entering or leaving it. It is because the neck serves as an important entry and exit point for such traversing viscera that an injury to these structures may make its manifestations at a site well away from the neck itself. A prime example is paralysis in the distal upper limb following a severe injury to the elements of the brachial plexus in the lower region of the neck.

The neck is a dangerously exposed area and the vital structures that pass through it are at greater risk than similar vital structures elsewhere (the brain is confined in the rigid shell of the skull, the heart and the lungs are encased in a bony thorax, and so on). Obvious evolutionary adaptations have resulted in a greater mobility of the cervical spine at the expense of safety. But because of fast protective reflexes, the neck is usually well defended in a conscious person. The exposed neck also allows for a quick access to the deeper structures such as to the trachea for an emergency tracheostomy and to the bleeding vessels for haemostasis on either side. Nevertheless, it is surprising to see considerable neglect of such life-saving procedures, perhaps because of the dramatic nature in which neck injury presents itself.

The extent of the injuries may range from transection of the cord without any obvious surface lesion to major laceration of the soft tissues producing major visible haemorrhage or respiratory distress.

A good working knowledge of the regional anatomy of the neck is essential in correlating the injury to the lesion produced.

2 Zones of the Neck

Conventionally, the neck has been divided into three zones for a better understanding of regional trauma (see Fig. 2.1).[2]

- Zone I starts from the medial infraclavicular part of the neck and extends to just below the cricoid cartilage and includes the related upper anterior mediastinum. It is also known as the region of the thoracic outlet. The contents include the proximal carotid arteries, the subclavian vessels, major vessels in the upper mediastinum, uppermost parts of the lungs and the viscera of the neck (oesophagus, trachea and the thoracic duct).

- Zone II includes the area from just above the cricoid cartilage to the angle of the jaw. This area sustains the maximum number of injuries mainly because it is the largest and the most unprotected part of the neck.

- Zone III is the small area of the neck between the angle of the mandible and the base of the skull and includes the maxillofacial region and the adjacent region of the skull.

The apprpriate management of neck injuries requires a concise understanding of the pathogenesis of neck trauma, based on which intelligent predictions can be made of the progression and outcome of most lesions. Not all of the clinical features are evident on presentation. Therefore, it is only with a sound knowledge of the mechanism and pathogenesis of neck injuries that the clinician can construct an overall picture of the extent of manifest and foreseeable damage, and plan an appropriate therapeutic and preventive management.

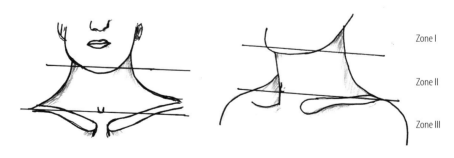

Zones of neck injury

Fig. 2.1

Presently most injuries to the neck are caused by road traffic accidents (RTA) or criminal violence (knife or gunshot wounds) and broadly speaking, the surface appearance may or may not indicate the cause of the trauma and the extent of the deeper injury.

Management of neck injuries requires immediate attention to the following important principles.

- *Firstly*, the ventilation must be protected. Tracheal injuries or injuries to the laryngopharynx need attention by way of careful and gentle endotracheal intubation or early tracheostomy before swelling makes these procedures difficult.

- *Secondly*, on-going haemorrhage should be stopped and potential haemorrhage prevented.

- *Thirdly*, injuries to cervical spine or cervical cord must be recognised. A delay in this diagnosis may result in an iatrogenic damage during subsequent handling or transportation. An incomplete cord transection may easily become a total transection with hyperextension of the cervical spine, for instance during intubation or rough handling at the medical facility.

2.1 Zone I

Zone I injuries (RTA crush or gunshot wounds) can result in major mediastinal haemorrhage, the control of which may require a speedy sternotomy or clavicular osteotomy. In this region, injuries of the oesophagus and trachea can result in acute mediastinitis and are difficult to control without adequate thoracotomy. Sometimes these injuries are concealed (or slow to develop) and are missed during initial assessment. A high index of suspicion is essential. Diagnostic angiography and venography should be considered in addition to routine radiological (chest and spine) and scanning procedures in patients with penetrating injury to the neck.[3]

Gastrografin oesophagography, oesophagoscopy and bronchoscopy should be given serious consideration in evaluating the full nature of suspect injuries to the viscera of the neck and the chest. Sufficient observation time must be spent in the absence of current signs or symptoms to exclude delayed manifestations.

2.2 Zone II

In the majority of cases zone II injuries must be explored surgically when the depth is deeper than platysma. Anterior injuries can damage carotid vessels, the thyroid gland, jugular veins, the trachea and the oesophagus. In other words, if the midline is crossed by the injury then the injury must be explored. If there is any suspicion of visceral injuries (trachea, larynx, hypopharynx, oesophagus) then a panendoscopy must be performed or the injury must be explored in the absence of facilities for panendoscopy. Posterolateral injuries can damage the vertebral artery and adjacent elements of the brachial plexus. Bleeding is very difficult to control in this region.

2.3 Zone III

Zone III injuries can result in damage to the carotid tree and within the limited space surrounded by bones, haemorrhage is difficult to control and a resultant cerebral ischaemia difficult to reverse. Endoscopy of trachea, hypopharynx, larynx and oesophagus must be performed to exclude visceral injuries. Arteriography should be performed because many seemingly occult lesions produce disastrous delayed consequences. Exploration must be generous. If mobilisation under anaesthetic relaxation does not provide sufficient space then mandibular osteotomy, on some occasions, may need to be undertaken for extracranial vascular injuries. On-table arteriography should be available and performed if time and the patient's condition permit.[3]

3 General Features of Incised Neck Injuries

These may be caused by knife cuts, glass or similar sharp objects. For the sake of simplicity, only incised injuries caused by knife cuts and glass are discussed here.

3.1 Knife Injuries

Knife injuries usually present as clearly well-defined sharp wounds. As the extent is well demarcated, the signs and symptoms are fairly obvious and present immediately. As most stabs are fairly deep, associated concealed haemorrhage or an injury to an underlying viscus may also be present.

When compared with penetrating trauma caused by a gunshot injury, stab wounds are relatively benign in the absence of an injury to a major blood vessel or to a vital structure, but there are wide exceptions to this statement.

If the incisional neck injury has involved deeper structures, such as muscles, the injury assumes the characteristics of a punctured wound. (In this context, a punctured, sharp wound is comparable to a deeply penetrating injury from the long blade of a knife.) Some of the clinical features will then be delayed.

If the plane of the injury is superficial, the wound may bleed profusely. The superficial blood vessels relating to platysma tend to retract from the wound margins, therefore the edges continue to ooze. In many elective surgical procedures of the neck, surgeons are besieged with such oozing wound margins and it is a well-recognised practice to apply haemostats to the deeper aspects of the platysma, well away from the wound margin and to evert the tissue for a short while for coagulative haemostasis.

In addition to the platysmal vessels, many other small subcutaneous arteries, arterioles and veins tend to retract from the wound margins. Such retracted ends of blood vessels are not easily sealed with diathermy cautery, which indeed can very easily burn and damage the skin margins with bad cosmetic results. Haphazard ligature ties to these vessels can easily lead to distortion of the subcutaneous tissue eventually resulting in disfigurement. Mechanical compression for some time or careful fine ties can usually control most of these haemorrhages.

With incised knife injuries, because the wounds are usually superficial, the extent of the underlying haematoma is small. The vessels involved in the incisional injuries are musculocutaneous vessels, blood vessels relating to the thyroid and vessels relating to the deeper muscles of the neck. When the knife injury is deep and results in an "incisional" puncture, the overlapping muscles and deep tissues prevent egress of blood and a subjacent haematoma results.

On rare occasions, stab injuries can be fairly benign unless a vessel has been disrupted or an important viscus has been entered.[3] However, stab wounds are hardly ever confined to the neck alone. Usually, the intention of the assailant is to cause maximum disfigurement or a fatality, therefore neck injuries are often associated with craniofacial injuries as well. Criminal cut-throat injury is an exception. But during this, because of the capacity of the upper cervical spine to acutely flex over the third, fourth, fifth and sixth cervical vertebrae, the chin is generally in contact with the thyroid cartilage and therefore the level of the injury is usually below this particular area.

Sharp knife punctures of the neck can be fairly deep and are often fatal!

Non-fatal injuries exhibit considerable damage to the lateral structures of the neck more often than to the structures of the anterior triangle. The posterolateral aspect of the neck is injured more often than the anterior parts.

3.2 Incised Glass Injuries

Accidental injuries with sheet-glass or window-pane glass produce superficial cuts, but spikes of broken glass can produce a much deeper penetrating wound. Such punctures can be small in size on the surface and yet may produce major disruption in the deeper planes. There may be concealed injuries present, such as to the trachea, oesophagus, major vessels and so on. When patients present with *in situ* glass spikes, haphazard removal of the glass may make the original injury worse unless facilities exist for proper haemostasis (Figs 3.1). The plane of injury is best determined by the removal of the glass spike under vision in the operating theatre, under anaesthesia! Sometimes, an arterial puncture, temporarily sealed by clots and the penetrating glass, starts to bleed profusely on removal. This may require an urgent exploration by extending the wound or by making formal approaches to the proximal and the distal parts of the injured vessel.

With RTA injuries car laminated windscreens usually shatter causing injuries to the front-seat occupants. The driver or an unbelted passenger may pass through the windscreen, sustaining faciomaxillary and other injuries. Laminated glass is adhesively bonded intrinsically and the effect of the impact usually results in the glass shattering into pieces.

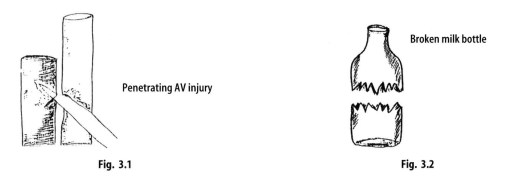

Penetrating AV injury

Fig. 3.1

Broken milk bottle

Fig. 3.2

The shattered windshield glass does not have as many sharp edges as shattered house-window glass. In respect of sharpness, the injuries are accordingly minimised.

The forward deceleration of an unrestrained driver or passenger during a RTA results in penetration through the windscreen and subsequent skull, face and neck injuries. The benefits of laminated glass windscreens and the use of proper seat-belts are obvious – fewer injuries are sustained! (see sections 4.4 and 5.3). In a series of 1042 cases, Schultz has emphasised windscreen injury to the facial region in decelerating front seat occupants of the car at an angle of approximately $45°$.[4] In his series most such injuries were superficial.

The major part of glass injuries involves the craniofacial region and the neck forms only a small part of the overall injury itself.

Another variety of the glass injury involves smashed bottle glass. The jagged ends of the bottle can produce gross disfiguring injuries of the face and the trunk (Fig. 3.2).

Bottle glass injuries are hardly ever fatal, but they often cause gross unsightly maxillofacial scars (Fig. 3.3). Such neck injuries are uncommon in isolation. They usually occur in conjunction with craniofacial and chest injuries. The victim tries to ward off the attacks and may thus sustain injuries to the hands as well.

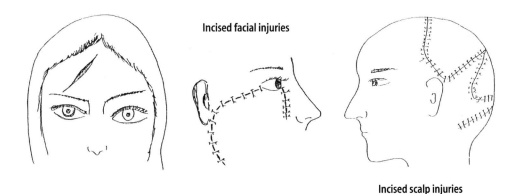

Incised facial injuries

Incised scalp injuries

Fig. 3.3

Lead-containing glass may be sufficiently radio-opaque to be visible on routine soft tissue X-ray. There is considerable medico-legal significance attached to such X-rays prior to undertaking repairs of facial wounds.

3.3 Management of Incised Neck Injuries

The emphasis of management is to treat or prevent airway obstruction, to provide haemostasis and to treat and prevent post-traumatic neurospinal injuries. The management includes a quick assessment of the vital signs; if these are stable then one should assess the peripheral structures for features of remote injury. An example being an injury to the brachial plexus in the neck, produced by a glass spike or knife, revealed by a proper neurological examination. Such examinations can only be postponed if the resultant delay in providing resuscitation endangers the patient. A high degree of suspicion is necessary to be able to avert such disasters. For instance, in relevant cases, a cautious and careful transportation of the patient with appropriate splints and supports can avoid further injuries to the roots of the brachial plexus or to the cervical spinal cord.

Following a generalised assessment the wound is examined from a haemostatic point of view. Most of the incised injuries tend to stop bleeding with simple and gentle manual compression with gauze or cotton wool. An arterial spurt is an obvious exception that indicates a severe extent of the injury and therefore special procedures need to be undertaken.

Major neck injuries can only be assessed properly in the environment of an operating theatre. Exploration has now become the mainstay of proper management in severe or deep injuries of the neck.

Minor superficial injuries (when no deeper structure is involved), should be closed cosmetically, utilising either subcuticular non-absorbable sutures, clips or "Steristrips". Since the incised injuries usually have well defined and well preserved apposing margins, a good primary repair results in the least amount of scarring and disfigurement.

If the injury appears to suggest a deeper damage, then an appropriate formal exploration must be performed. In presence of a neurovascular lesion or signs and symptoms of visceral damage, it would be entirely wrong to close the skin or to undertake such an exploration under a local anaesthetic. Following a thorough evaluation of the patient, proper exploration and primary repair should be undertaken under a formal general anaesthetic. An exploration may necessitate extending the wound so that the injury can be managed more thoroughly.

A punctured wound is very difficult to assess from a superficial examination because the extent is variable and the sandwiching layers of the muscle and soft tissue overlap the actual puncture track. It follows therefore that whereas a superficially incised wound can be extended in the same plane for a proper inspection, a punctured wound should not be explored at the same depth for fear of causing a comparable iatrogenic damage or missing a significant injury altogether. Preferably, a separate access should be used for a proper exploration, reaching to the depths of the primary injury.

Wounds have to be treated on merit but also on principle; incised wounds can be assessed relatively easily and can be repaired by primary suturing. Cosmetic considerations must be borne in mind during such a repair.

If time and the patient's condition allows it, a pre-operative photographic documentation of such injuries is very useful especially where cosmetic considerations are involved.

4 General Features of Lacerated Neck Injuries

Lacerated injuries to the neck are usually caused by road traffic accidents (RTA) or by criminal activities. The incidence is obviously different in the urban and in the rural areas (see sections 12 and 13).

Lacerated criminal injuries can be caused by a knife, a glass or a gun, but these can also be produced (although rarely) by a blunt assault resulting in tissue disruption.

Accidental lacerated injuries are commonly produced by RTAs, but can also be produced by falls. Blunt trauma of RTA impact, the shearing effects of dragging on the road, friction injury, puncture by foreign bodies such as grit and stones, can all act on the tissue to produce a laceration.

In general, the commonest cause of lacerated injuries to the neck are RTAs, but lacerated wounds of the neck form only a small part of the overall injuries sustained by the victim in an RTA.

Puncture injuries to the neck caused by spikes etc are rare. Behaviourally these are deep lacerated injuries and are grossly infected.

Penetration of deeper tissue by any foreign body, including a knife, infects the wound and transfers surface contaminants within.

4.1 Lacerated Injuries Caused by Knife or Glass

Most of these injuries are multiple. Windscreen injuries produce various cuts and bruises and, occasionally, cause laceration of the neck, but neck injuries in this context hardly ever occur in isolation. When injuries are caused by bottle glass or a knife, then these are deep, multiple and infected.

Lacerated injuries caused by a knife are deeper than those caused by glass and therefore can easily injure the neurovascular structures and the viscera of the neck.

4.2 General Features and Ballistics of Gunshot Injuries to the Neck

Firearms used in criminal activities include the following.[5]

- *Handguns*. These may be single-shot pistols, derringers (similar to single-shot pistols, but with multiple barrels), revolvers or auto-loading pistols (semi-automatics). These are easy to carry, small, pocket-sized but are generally not very powerful.

- *Rifles*. The bores of these weapons are rifled. They have a minimum barrel length of 16 inches. They can be of single-shot type or work as repeaters using lever action, pump action or auto-loading mechanisms.

- *Shotguns*. These are smooth-bore firearms with a minimum barrel length of 18 inches. When sawn off, they act as explosive pistols. These are usually double-barrelled and use cartridges containing pellets. The pellets spread out and the extent, but not the depth, of the injury is large.

- *Submachine guns*. These are machine pistols with a rifled bore and fire pistol ammunition. These are auto-repeaters with injury potential ranging usually between pistols and rifles. They can be concealed as long pistols and can be fitted on wooden casings to elongate the operational length for ease of use.

- *Machine guns*. These are rifled repeaters, high powered and have a high injury-potential. They are lightweight and use a loaded magazine or a strip of bullets.

A typical bullet has a cartridge case containing 70% copper and 30% zinc; although less common varieties can be made of steel.

The bullet acts as a pointed missile and enters the body in a linear trajectory, although some circular motion is involved initially. Because the softness of the neck offers much less resistance than the other parts of the body, many high velocity missiles cause death by going through the neck and emerging from the other side.

Isolated rifle injuries to the neck are extremely uncommon and are very often fatal. Rifle injuries to other parts of the body are much more common. Non-fatal rifle injuries produce deep damage. An important consideration with a rifle bullet is the possibility of the bullet traversing to the vertebral bodies and then ricocheting away, either in the reverse direction or as is more likely, in another direction, emerging out of the neck from a wound well away from or close to the wound of entry.

The ricocheting path of the bullet produces additional damage (Fig. 4.1). The injury is deep and when the bullet strikes the surface of the skin, depending on its velocity, the thermal effects "sterilise" the superficial structures. This "sterility" is associated with cauterisation of the wound track. The neck is an exposed part of the body, but when it is covered by a garment, the ragged pieces of the fabric can be dragged in, as a foreign body, into the deeper parts of the neck. Although the initial passage of the bullet may thermally "sterilise" the

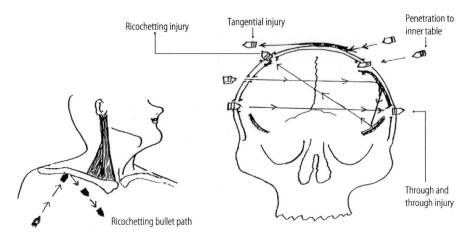

Fig. 4.1

tissue, as will be seen later, subsequent events (cavitations, and so on) may immediately contaminate the wound (see section 4.2.4).

The rifle bullet wound is technically a puncture-laceration in which the wound of entry is deceptively very small, although the depth of the injury is usually fairly substantial. The exit wound is much more disorganised and everted (Fig. 4.2) depending on the shape of the bullet or more accurately, the frontal areas of the bullet mass. A sharp and conical missile disrupts less tissue particles whereas a less streamlined projectile, with its blunted or flatter profile will have a mushrooming effect destroying and fragmenting more tissue.

The terminal energy imparted to the tissue by the bullet determines the injury potential. A .22 is eight times as powerful in releasing this terminal energy as a .38 revolver.

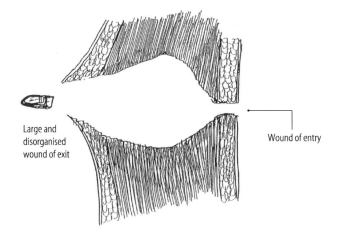

Fig. 4.2

There is very little generalised superficial trauma present. The superficial appearance can be deceptive and may mislead the clinician into assuming that deeper structures are not involved. A good assessment and a high degree of suspicion are necessary. No bullet wound must be accepted as a trivial injury, no matter how benign it looks superficially.

The bullet itself may not cause a great deal of harm, unless, of course, its trajectory includes an important structure which gets damaged by track disruption, shock-wave compression, laceration or puncture by the fragmented bone travelling as a secondary missile.[6]

In most cases of neck injury, a guarded initial conservative approach yields better results. A methodical assessment is a prerequisite to preparing a plan of action. This is essential. It is wrong to embark on a blind exploration without orderly preoperative assessment, unless it is a life-threatening situation.

The clinical behaviour and pathogenesis of bullet injuries are related to the mass of the bullet and to the velocity with which it is travelling. The mass (weight) of the bullet (detachable lead missile) is easily determined by the following formula:[7]

$$WT - WR$$

where WT is the total weight of the bullet and WR is the residual weight of the bullet complex after firing.

The velocity of the bullet is dependent on

● the firing capacity of the firearm

● the distance from which the firearm has been fired

● the size or the mass of the charge contained in the bullet substance.

Generally, firearms capable of generating a missile (bullet) velocity of more than 2500 feet/s are referred to as high-powered or high-velocity weapons.[3]

A great deal of the force of the bullet is lost in dissipating the tissue in various directions. The destruction of the tissue is proportional to the energy of the bullet with which the tissue is destroyed, dispersed and disintegrated in various directions.

The kinetic energy (EK) of a bullet can be obtained from the following formula

$$EK = \frac{M \times V^2}{2}$$

where M is the mass of the bullet and V is the velocity of the bullet.

It can be seen from this equation that even a relatively small change in the velocity can make a considerable difference in the energy produced by the bullet itself. Here lies the difference between pistol and rifle bullet injuries.

However, not all of the force of the bullet is responsible for the tissue damage. In other words, when the bullet leaves the body (exits), the unused energy (with which the bullet leaves the body) is not utilised for tissue destruction. The tissue is only damaged by the wounding energy of the bullet.

The wounding energy (*EW*) of a bullet can be calculated from the following formula:

$$EW = EK_{entry} - EK_{exit}$$

where EK_{entry} is the kinetic energy at the wound of entry, and EK_{exit} is the residual kinetic energy at the site of the exit of the bullet from the wound.

The wounding energy is necessarily less than the kinetic energy of the bullet.

As a bullet leaves a gun, the air resistance slows it down absorbing some of the force. A typical streamlined projectile travels with minimal resistance until it touches the skin and the deeper tissue. The frontal pointed end is resisted by the tissue slowing the velocity down. The bullet's centre of gravity rotates from the rear of the bullet to its front and in doing so creates a tumble. The bullet still moves forward but now presenting a broader frontal profile. This will disrupt more tissue making a larger tunnel and increasing the secondary missile effect. If the bullet is fragmented then the fragments will transmit their energies in various directions, enlarging the tunnel and producing a widespread damage by tissue displacement. When the bullet travels through the tissue, four different changes occur and the following effects are produced:

- local track formation
- secondary missile effect
- remote shock-wave effect
- temporary cavitation effect.

4.2.1 Local Track Formation

As the bullet passes through the tissue, depending on its shape and the trajectory, a tunnel (track) is created with loss of tissue substance. The tissue is lost because it has been pushed away, vaporised or has been dragged out by the bullet (Fig. 4.3).

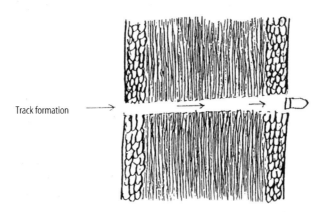

Track formation

Fig. 4.3

If the shape of the bullet is conical or cigar shaped, with the pointed end at its front (as is typical with most bullets), then the wound of entry is fairly neat and small, and the path of the track is fairly straight, but the path does increase in width and diameter as the bullet approaches the exit wound.

Closer to the exit wound, the bullet disrupts a greater proportion of tissue and the marginal area is avulsed out violently with general loss of the adjoining tissue. In other words, there is typically a greater destruction of the tissue at the exit.

If the shape of the bullet is such that the conical frontal end is replaced by a slightly flattened one, as is seen with the so-called "dumdum" bullet, then the track will be much wider and more tissue will be destructed from the impact and thus a so-called "mushrooming" effect will be produced.[8] If the bullet has been fired by a low-velocity weapon (pistol or revolver), then the track itself is the main area of injury and fewer other injuries of significance are produced.

4.2.2 Secondary Missile Effects

During its passage through the track the bullet encounters tissues of different densities, such as tough inelastic fibrous tissue, muscle fibres and bone. Such tissues are torn off and the dissipating force from the kinetic energy of the travelling bullet shoots these tiny pieces off in multiple trajectories as "secondary missiles". The overall damage is therefore scattered over a much wider area. Such a secondary missile effect is more commonly seen with bones, rather than with muscle fibres. Bone fragments, if large, may act like a "dumdum" bullet (Figs 4.4 and 4.5).

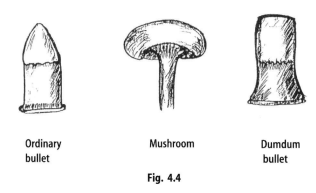

Ordinary bullet   Mushroom   Dumdum bullet

Fig. 4.4

4.2.3 Remote Shock-wave Effects

As the bullet passes through the track, it displaces adjacent tissue hydraulically. If the tissue is water logged, a greater hydraulic disturbance will be produced. These hydraulic shock

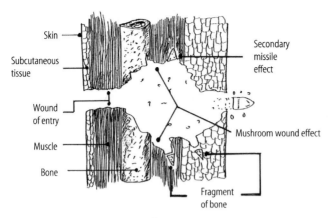

Fig. 4.5

waves can be transmitted over a long distance and can damage a remote structure intrinsically. If there is a nerve in the path of this shock wave, such shock waves can disrupt axons leaving the epineurial sheath intact. Such shock waves are exaggerated if the tissue has air or gas present in addition to water (urinary bladder and hollow organs of the gastrointestinal tract).

Occasionally, with bomb blasts, a shrapnel or bomb fragment travelling close to the anterior abdominal wall, may produce shock waves of enough intensity to produce gastrointestinal perforations while the anterior abdominal wall may remain intact. The same may apply to the neck in relation to the viscera of the neck.

4.2.4 Temporary Cavitation Effects

As the bullet makes a tunnel and tissue is pushed out from the track, cavitation is produced. Such a cavitation is proportional to the wounding energy and to the amount of energy transferred from the bullet to the side walls of the cavity (Fig. 4.6).

Cavitation effect is seen frequently with bullets travelling over 300 m/s. As the velocity increases, this cavitation effect becomes more intense. At 600 m/s, cavitation is quite large and dramatic destruction of tissue occurs.

Whenever the travelling velocity is greater than 100 m/s, although the track may be quite small, the overall diameter of the cavity may be 30 times the diameter of the missile. A large amount of tissue is disrupted from this cavitation effect in the immediate vicinity of the track.

High water content produces more cavitation damage. Proportionately less damage occurs in tissues containing elastic fibres, such as lungs and skin.

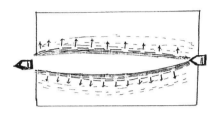

Cavitation effect

Fig. 4.6

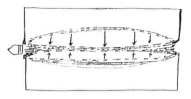

Reversed cavitation effect

Fig. 4.7

Once maximum cavitation has occurred, a few milliseconds later, the cavity collapses back to the size of the local track, and with this reciprocal phenomenon there is a great vacuum produced in the suddenly reducing cavity. This results in sucking in (into the wound), of foreign bodies, microorganisms and so forth. This explains the high proportion of infection seen with high-velocity bullet wounds even though the thermal and the vibratory energy of the bullet may be expected to have "sterilised" the area of the track (Fig. 4.7).

A wound that has been cavitated and has resulted in greater disruption, must be surgically treated and decontaminated. Those antibiotics which have a greater access to the necrotic area and which achieve a greater blood level in a shorter space of time, should be used liberally, such as aminoglycoside, cephalosporin, etc.

In general, debridement of the wound should be done within the first 6 hours and all severely damaged tissue should be removed. A relatively more radical approach is needed for damaged subcutaneous tissues, muscles and viscera. Less radical excision is required in skin, tendon, fascia and bone. Antibiotics and protection against tetanus must be provided.

The whole track of the wound should be debrided.

4.3 General Features of Shotgun Injury of the Neck

A shotgun is a long smooth-bored barrelled gun. The cartridge used for firing is not very large. The proximal portion of the cartridge contains an explosive charge which lies around a cap into which is attached a primer. Beyond this, within the paper or the plastic cartridge, is a pack of wad or wadding (Fig. 4.8).

The wad is in close contact with a more distal compartment which is filled with small shots or pellets. The pellets range from 2 to 4 mm in diameter. A general cartridge contains approximately 300 such pellets (range 90–585 cl.).

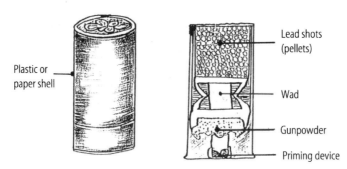

Plastic or paper shell

Lead shots (pellets)

Wad

Gunpowder

Priming device

Fig. 4.8

Shotgun injuries are hardly ever confined to the neck, because at the usual distance from where these are fired, the adjacent parts of the face and chest are inevitably involved.

Criminal shotgun injuries almost always involve the craniofacial region and are often fatal. Treatment of survivors of close range injuries is very difficult because different structures in different planes are injured.

A short-range shotgun trauma, such as from 5 m or less, delivers a considerable energy to the wound and in this regard the transmission of force compares well with the transmission of force seen in a bullet wound caused by a high-velocity firearm, such as a high-powered rifle.

Shotgun pellets spread out from the barrel, travelling in an inverted conical fashion. As the pellets fan out, the force is dissipated and with the increase in the distance, the momentum and therefore the wounding energy of each pellet are considerably reduced. Some fragmentation takes place of the pellets as the pellets travel through the air. The mass is reduced due to fragmentation and the momentum is accordingly reduced. The air resistance also slows down the pellets. Tissue being a medium denser than air, penetration through skin reduces the amount of energy transfer and therefore the velocity.

Most of the serious shotgun wounds are produced from a range of 20 m or less, beyond which the force is not sufficient to inflict any major damage, except perhaps, to the eyes (Fig. 4.9).

From a far distance (greater than 20 m), the spread of the multidirectional pellets results in superficial injuries to the entire body including the face, the neck, chest and the abdomen.

A shotgun injury caused from a 10 m distance, usually penetrates, but does not pass through strong muscles, therefore most of the pellets remain trapped in the sheath of the muscles (Fig. 4.10).

Shotgun injuries are particularly nasty if they have been caused at close range. The pellets enter and penetrate the skin in a limited area, producing a tremendous amount of crush against deeper tissues, which they are unable to penetrate.

A neck injury caused by a shotgun blast at a distance less than 5 m is almost always fatal. In rare survivors, multiple injuries due to fragmentation (secondary missile effects) are present. Serious neurospinal injuries or delayed secondary aneurysm formation may occur.

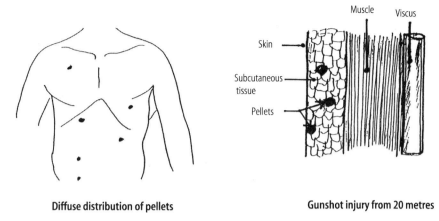

Diffuse distribution of pellets · Gunshot injury from 20 metres

Fig. 4.9

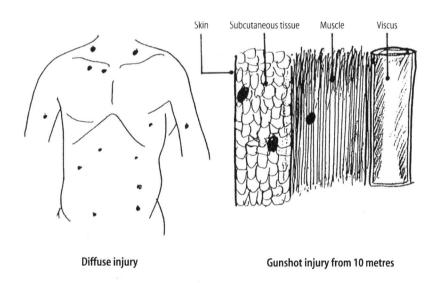

Diffuse injury · Gunshot injury from 10 metres

Fig. 4.10

Maceration relates not only to superficial muscles but also to the sandwiched neurovascular structures and to nearby viscera of the neck. The damage usually occurs at multiple levels, to a small area, and the only hope for salvage is immediate surgical intervention.

Close-range injury is almost always fatal and only a small minority of victims survive this trauma. The appearance of this type of injury is a mixture of compression, burns and fragmentation (Fig. 4.11). Such an injury is a very aggressive criminal injury. Here the majority of the pellets strike the victim; few being lost to the exterior! The pellets possess

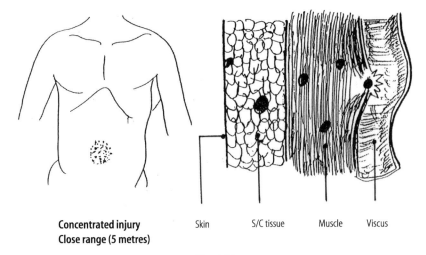

Concentrated injury   Skin   S/C tissue   Muscle   Viscus
Close range (5 metres)

Fig. 4.11

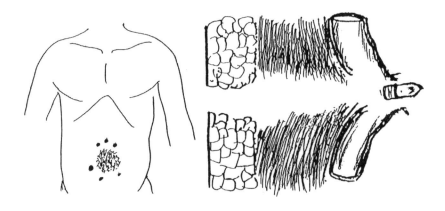

Total disruption similar to rifle bullet injury
concentrated close range (1 metre) injury

Fig. 4.12

sufficient force to penetrate the structures deeper than muscles (Fig. 4.11) and some pellets may enter the spinal cord.

In wounds caused by a shotgun fired at a distance of 1 m or less (attempted suicide) there is a large central defect present measuring 3–6 cm in diameter with a surrounding halo of pellets (Fig. 4.12).

Severe maceration and disruption of the area occurs with such a wound, usually causing immediate death. In the unusual circumstance of the shotgun neck injury missing vital structures, there is sufficient tissue maceration to produce severe bleeding and contamination.

The wadding, paper or plastic parts of the cartridge may act as foreign bodies in the depths of the wound, in close-range shotgun injuries.

The shorter the distance, the more the transfer of thermal energy to the wound site. In contact wounds, abundant skin and subcutaneous burn is present. Such flash burns are the forensic hallmark of close-range shotgun injuries.

4.3.1 Management Priorities of Shotgun Injuries to the Neck

The first priority is the preservation of respiration and therefore an early consideration must be given to either a prolonged endotracheal intubation or to a preliminary tracheostomy (which is more useful).

The second consideration relates to haemostasis and vascular salvage. Immediate and effective haemostasis can only be achieved in the operating theatre. This should be combined with fast and adequate blood volume restoration.

Management of visceral and neurological damage are the subsequent priorities requiring independent actions on merit.

Even when the shotgun has been fired from a long distance (more than 20 m), some pellets may penetrate the softer parts of the face producing generalised damage.

In the region of the neck, the tissue being fairly soft, the pellets can enter underneath the platysma and may be lodged at the depth of the sternomastoid and scalene muscles. The roots of the brachial plexus, superficial blood vessels of the neck such as the external jugular vein and the veins relating to the thyroid can be injured. Pellets can enter the larynx and severe injury can be caused to the laryngeal mass or to the vessels and the regional nerves (such as the recurrent laryngeal nerves and the vagi).

As few as one or two pellets penetrating the carotid sheath may cause a substantial damage. Frequent physical examinations and arteriographic evaluation are necessary in such wounds to exclude such vascular injuries. If such a critical degree of expectant observation is not possible then urgent exploration must be undertaken.

A shotgun range of 10 m makes it difficult to remove all of the pellets and X-ray evaluation, particularly depth views and lateral views, may be necessary to locate these radio-opaque foreign bodies.

Approximately half (40–65%) of penetrating neck injuries present with clinical features warranting exploration. Of these 35–40% need therapeutic surgery.[8]

4.4 Road Traffic Accident Lacerations

Injuries to vehicle occupants constitute the predominant cause of motor vehicle crash deaths. In recent years in the UK, almost 70% of all RTA-related deaths were due to people injured as occupants of vehicles such as cars, light trucks and vans. Pedestrian deaths represent the second largest category of motor vehicle deaths.[9]

Injuries to pedestrians can be caused by a direct hit by the main body of the car, its door handles, decorations and trimming or due to crushing against another vehicle. Crushing and lacerating injuries are caused in this way, although neck injuries are much less frequent than limb injuries.

Even blunt injuries to the neck in road accidents can produce lacerations by direct impact, decelerating, rotary and shearing forces. In fact, a variety of such forces act together to produce overall vehicular injuries.[3,10]

In many car-manufacturing countries of the world it has become illegal to install hazardous car decorations which could be potentially harmful to a pedestrian victim. (Car monograms have either been abandoned or are being made in a collapsible form; the collapsible Mercedes Benz and Rolls Royce insignia are examples). Unfortunately the fixing of car decorations is only regulated in car-manufacturing countries, but in many places, road safety or vehicle safety considerations are not always given due prominence. Harmful car decorations are secondarily installed, such as flashy bumpers, protruding fenders, unregulated spoilers, chariot-style tyre rims, resulting in major lacerated injuries to the pedestrians. Neck injuries from such objects are very rare in isolation, and if and when these occur to pedestrians, the chances of survival are greatly reduced.

Following an RTA, multiple injuries are much more common than isolated injuries of the neck. More often than not, injuries are present elsewhere, such as to the head, chest, abdomen or the limbs. RTA-related neck injuries cause more damage to drivers than to front-seat passengers.

Within the car, the rear-seat unrestrained occupants may sustain impact neck injuries when they decelerate forward against the head rests on the front seats.

Front-seat occupants usually sustain injuries as a result of shattering glass or as a result of hitting various internal parts of the car such as the dashboard, rear-view mirror, steering wheel or door frame.[3,10]

Arterial lacerations of the neck sometimes occur in public transport vehicles, such as coaches, buses or trains. Such wounds are usually dirty with an abundance of soiling and there may be foreign bodies present. Lacerated wounds of the neck are difficult to treat and they are often very dangerous. Vascular injuries in these situations are almost always associated with additional major non-vascular injuries. These injuries must be assessed in the context of overall damage, but preservation of the cardiorespiratory status takes priority. A proper assessment can only be made in the operating theatre. Prior to operating, it is essential to assess and then to document, injuries relating to the neurovascular structures and also to the neck viscera. An important late legal consideration is "Has the final lesion been produced by the injury, careless transportation or by the exploratory operation?". Unguarded or haphazard neck exploration may totally sever a partially injured nerve root. An uninjured thoracic duct may be inadvertently damaged during a hurried exploration. Partial spinal cord transection may become complete during transportation or endotracheal intubation.

Protection against tetanus must be provided. To a previously immunised patient, a booster dose of toxoid suffices. To an non-immunised low-risk patient following initial antitetanus toxoid administration, a full course (booster at 6 weeks and 6 months) must be recommended. To a high-risk patient with major contamination, antitetanus serum, duly skin tested, should be given, followed by active immunisation with toxoid.

4.5 Puncture Injuries of the Neck

Other than those caused by knives, firearms or glass, puncture injuries of the neck are rare, but can be caused in road accidents. Criminal injuries have been known to be caused by metal spikes such as iron rods, cricket wickets, wooden fencing spikes and so on.

Behaviourally these types of wounds produce deep lacerations and transmit considerable force to the penetrated and the crushed areas. By definition, the wound of entry is a small inverted puncture whose margins become ragged, irregular and everted on removal of the spike. Such injuries are usually badly contaminated and infection is present from the outset. Since the object causing the injury is large, it follows that the depth of the injury would most certainly be smaller than knife injuries. Puncture knife injuries to the neck are usually deep. Cut-throat injuries are traditionally slicing incised injuries.

A puncture wound is difficult to assess from a cursory examination. The sandwiching layers of muscle and subcutaneous tissue afford temporary overlapping cover and a deeper injury may remain unrecognised. Formal exploration is therefore necessary. This variety of wound is very deceptive and may result in a major life-threatening injury within a seemingly innocent-looking wound of entry. Temporary initial haemostasis can usually be achieved with extrinsic compression followed by formal exploration and repair. A good and reliable airway must be maintained. Since the wound is basically infected, protection against tetanus must also be provided, in addition to antibiotics.

In recent years, an aggressive management strategy involving early exploration has been recommended in all types of neck puncture wounds.[8] This, of course, presupposes an adequate preoperative assessment, which is as complete as time and the patient's condition permit.

5 General Features of Crush and Closed Injuries of the Neck

In this complex group are clustered those varied neck injuries in which a severe force is applied to a small local area resulting in superficial and deep damage.

Crushing can occur from falling industrial machinery or by car collisions. The result is tissue compression and violent disruption. The skin and subcutaneous tissue may shear.

Maceration effect, as it happens in limbs with crush syndrome, does not occur in the neck. Whatever the direction of the crushing force, the immediate dangers are asphyxia from laryngotracheal compression and vascular obstruction. Both these problems are life threatening. For these reasons, most industrial compressions and accidental crush injuries of the neck are usually fatal. Survivors exhibit many kinds of soft tissue trauma, including surgical emphysema, mediastinitis from oesophageal perforation and so on. Respiratory salvage and haemostasis are prime considerations in the management.

The most common examples of crush neck injuries are seen in high-speed road traffic accidents (RTAs) on motorways. In a multiple car collision, death can occur from violent mechanical crush of the neck, multiple injuries and injuries of the neck that can produce asphyxiation.

The most prevalent examples of closed injuries of the neck are seen in car accidents when the front seats are not fitted with head rests. "Closed" injuries are internal injuries of the neck produced in the absence of an external injury. An important example in this group is the whiplash injury to the cervical spinal cord (see section 26).

5.1 Crush Injuries of the Neck Caused by a Blunt Assault

As the usual intention of an assailant is to cause maximum damage and facial disfigurement these injuries are inflicted mostly to the skull and to the maxillofacial region. The neck in such situations is an unintended bystander! Neck injuries are produced only in association with such intended damage.

A blunt injury caused by club, truncheon, fist or boxing glove may result in fracture of the cervical spine if applied from the posterolateral or posterior directions (see section 26).

Anterior injuries to the neck may result in laryngeal fracture or tracheal injuries (see sections 31 and 32). Blunt injuries of this nature are associated with considerable haematoma and there are usually additional associated injuries present in the region of the face, the skull and also of the chest.

Major blunt injuries to the neck usually result in a tremendous amount of haematoma and also injury to the deeper structures. An example of blunt assault also includes attempted strangulation, when the extent of the injury could range from surface bruising and haematoma to asphyxia and local damage to the laryngopharynx.

Management depends on the severity of the injury. Preservation of respiration is of prime importance. Tracheostomy or cricothyroidostomy may have to be undertaken urgently before oedema or haematoma masks the landmarks, making these interventions more difficult and hazardous.

5.2 Crush Injuries Produced by Industrial Trauma

Industrial crush injuries to the neck presuppose presence of limb injuries as well. If the limbs were unaffected then the compression could be relieved by moving the compressing object from the neck area. Crush injuries to the skin are caused by pinching or squeezing of the skin between two blunt surfaces. Post-traumatic infection is very common.

Industrial compression injuries to the neck are very frequently fatal because of asphyxia and associated crush fracture of the skull or of the maxillofacial region. Patients are usually unconscious and may exhibit respiratory embarrassment. The crushing objects should be removed quickly and the airway maintained. Nasotracheal intubation or cricothyroidostomy is usually necessary, to be substituted later, with formal tracheostomy. Injuries to deep structures are then reassessed before definitive treatment can begin elsewhere.

5.3 Crush Injuries of the Neck Caused by Road Traffic Accidents

These constitute the largest number of crush injuries to the region of the neck. In these, the element of sustained compression results in aggravation of the initial damage. There is a considerable maceration of the deeper tissues and there are many uncontrolled bleeding sites present. As haemostatic circumferential compression of the neck is not possible, most such crush injuries are immediately fatal, since haemorrhage cannot be adequately and quickly controlled as in the periphery.

Non-fatal RTA injuries to the neck also include additional skull, maxillofacial and chest injuries. An example of such road accidents is the trapping of rear-seat passengers in the confined space between the front and the rear seats of the car. The front-seat occupants also suffer from similar trauma, such as the driver pushed against the driving wheel of the car and the front-seat passenger trapped in the twisted seat in the front compartment. The only hope of salvage is immediate surgery.

There is a tremendous difficulty in transporting patients who have sustained compression/crush injuries to the neck in RTAs. They may be unconscious and suffocation may already have been produced either as a result of tracheal damage or as a result of spreading emphysema, haematoma, or aspiration. Such patients may also suffer from hypovolaemic or cardiogenic shock and therefore should be resuscitated urgently.

A medical rescue squad ("Rescue Team" in the UK or "Flying Squad" in the USA) assisted by the fire and rescue service (who can cut through car frames and doors) equipped with an on-site operating theatre, is the only sure way of reducing fatality rates. Such rescue teams should stay on call near major motorways or highways.

In RTAs, crushing or pressure forces are frequently accompanied by shearing forces that may lead to stripping of large areas of skin, subcutaneous tissue and muscles and their vascular pedicles, from trunk and limbs.[11]

RTA crush injuries to the neck may result in vascular and non-vascular lesions. Vascular lesions are more common than one would expect.

Table 5.1 shows an estimate by the American Association for Automotive Medicine describing various types of vascular injuries sustained in RTAs.

A similar series modified from Rich's *Vascular trauma*,[12] showed the following variation between civilian and military injuries related to blood vessels (see Table 5.2).

Table 5.1 Various vascular injuries sustained in RTAs (American Association for Automotive Medicine)

Vascular wall defects (lacerations)	51.4%
Transection of vessels	38.2%
Arteriovenous fistula (puncture)	6.9%
Arterial spasm	0.8%
Intimal flap (dissections)	Negligble

Table 5.2 Variation between civilian and military injuries related to blood vessels

Injury	Civilian (%)	Military (%)
Laceration	51.4	56.0
Transection	38.2	40.0
Puncture	6.9	0
Contusion	2.7	4.0
Spasm	0.8	0
Total	100.0	100.0

Reproduced with permission from *Surg Clin N Am* **53**: 1367–92, 1973.

5.4 Closed Injuries of the Neck

For most closed injuries of the neck the causative mechanism is a posterior blunt trauma to the region of the cervical spine or to the laryngopharyngeal area anteriorly and, accordingly, such injuries are often associated with neurogenic shock and respiratory arrest.

A common variety of closed neck injury is whiplash of the cervical spine. During the deceleration experienced in a car accident, the driver decelerates forward until restrained by the seat-belt or, if unbelted, the steering wheel, and then, because of a reflex action, recoils backwards. During such a recoil manoeuvre, the cervical spine is extended backwards in its upper part and flexed forwards in its lower part. This is followed by reversed or exactly reciprocal movement resulting in severe transmission of force at the junction of the fixed to the mobile parts of the cervical vertebrae. Commonly this results in the maximum force being transmitted on to the odontoid process of the second cervical vertebra (axis). The odontoid process is securely entrapped in the ring of the first cervical vertebra (atlas), but following a whiplash injury, it can be fractured and disrupted producing a spinal cord damage such as transection (see section 26). Spinal shock precedes actual transection. Such injuries are comparable to those seen in judicial hanging where the vertebral disarticulation is preceded by spinal shock and then rupture of spinal cord. The neurogenic shock in this situation precedes cardiogenic shock and respiratory death.

Closed injuries of the neck are also associated with skull and face injuries that are caused by direct damage against the fixed structures of the car. Contrecoup intracranial injuries and fractures of the lateral ribs, are also fairly common in such situations. Such closed injuries, can also produce brachial plexus lesions by avulsing one or more roots of cervical nerves (C_5–T_1). Most neck-injured RTA survivors are unconscious and trapped within the vehicle.

Closed-neck injuries include carotid sheath injuries (see section 15). A violent blunt injury to the neck may result in acute thrombosis of the carotid artery or the internal jugular vein (see sections 15.4, 19 and 20.5). In rare cases the vagus nerve is similarly damaged (see section 25). Vasovagal shock and recurrent laryngeal nerve trauma may result from this injury.

RTA whiplashing of the cervical spine resulting in damage to the spinal cord can occur equally on racing circuits with high-performance cars as well as in family cars at normal travelling speeds. Rocket ejection-seat injuries (astronauts and combat aircraft pilots) can also result in deceleration injuries to the neck, in a similar fashion.

An important preventive aspect of RTA injuries has been the legally enforced introduction of seat-belts in cars. Modern car seat-belts are now of the inertia-reel type. This allows a gentle forward movement of the belted person, so that the normal activity of the driver and the normal movements of the front-seat passenger are not inconveniently restrained. The inertia reel is so designed that when sudden deceleration of the restrained person takes place (such as in an accident) then the seat-belt is immediately locked, entrapping the person at one particular place, preventing forward propulsion.[13,14]

With the awareness that a simple lap seat-belt was not useful in preventing blunt injuries of the head, neck and of the chest, the addition of the shoulder part of the seat-belt was introduced. The modern inertia seat-belt is a composite of a shoulder strap as well as a lap belt. Nevertheless at the time of crisis, when the body decelerates forwards and the inertia seat-belt is activated, the seat-belt is only capable of restraining the trunk, the abdomen and the pelvis (Fig. 5.1).

To the positive advantage of the belted person, relevant kinematic researches have shown that in comparison with the unrestrained person, the belted occupant's trajectory of

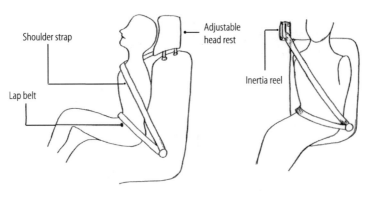

Fig. 5.1

deceleration is quite different when wearing a three-point lap and diagonal retractor seat-belt in a 30 mph frontal crash.[15] Such belts offer a definite overall protection and have dramatically reduced the incidence of personal injury in RTAs.

Despite the use of the modern seat-belts, whiplashing of the cervical spine is still possible and in order to minimise this, head rests have become compulsorily installed in modern cars. Unfortunately in many countries, legislative controls are poor and therefore either the head rests are removed or seat-belts are not installed at all. The involved clinician should therefore encourage the policy makers to install and to legally enforce the use of seat-belts and head rests. The combination of inertia lap-and-shoulder belts with head rests has resulted in dramatic reduction of the head and neck injuries previously associated with most car accidents.[15] Unfortunately, a small number of compression and avulsion injuries have recently come to light, having been caused by sudden compressive entrapment by modern seat-belts. Duodenal perforations, sternal fractures and colonic perforations are related to wearing of seat-belts. However, it must be clearly emphasised that the vast reduction of craniofacial, neck and other injuries that a seat-belt and a head rest can prevent fully justifies the use of the belt despite the very small percentage of belt-related injuries.

Apart from legislative penalties imposed on those who do not wear seat-belts, law courts in many countries take into account the wearing of seat-belts as an important matter in the settlement of personal injury claims. In awarding compensations for personal injury, British courts take into consideration whether the injured person (driver or passenger) had worn a seat-belt at the time of the accident. If the injured person had been restrained, then the court holds that all necessary precautions had been taken in order to avoid personal injury. If the driver or passenger had not worn the belt, then it is generally held that they had not fully taken all necessary conceivable precautions and any financial compensation is lessened so that the unbelted injured person shares the burden of liability.

Although the British government was among the first to publish details as to the usefulness of wearing seat-belts, the reaction of the British judiciary system was unexpectedly different. The judiciary held that it was a matter of civil liberty as to whether a car driver or passenger choose to wear a seat-belt. This choice was compared with personal freedoms such as with those related to voluntary abortions, attempted suicides and so on. It is only recently that in keeping with the European Union practices that laws have been introduced making the use of seat-belts compulsory.

In some countries, the wearing of seat-belts by rear seat occupants is also being legally enforced at the present time.

Although legislative reforms may take longer to implement in less well-developed countries the positive benefits of seat-belt use must be highlighted to law makers or magistrates of traffic courts. Such a positive encouragement in conjunction with better public education must be provided to achieve reduction of morbidity and mortality figures.

Patients with injuries to the cervical spine should not be transported injudiciously. A correct approach, if the initial diagnosis is of whiplash injury to the cervical spine, is to encase the patient's head and neck in a suitable splint so that during transport to the hospital, further injury of the spinal cord or of the viscera can be prevented. Such pneumatic and malleable splints are part of ambulance equipment in the UK and USA. A cervical collar is a cheap alternative that can be used anywhere.

The awareness of the safety-conscious community has led the policy makers to take notice of the kinematics of vehicle accidents and to devise laws relating to seat-belts, infant bucket seats, rear seat passenger seat-belts and so on. Increased public awareness has led to continuous improvements in the interior design of cars and the inclusion of many safety features. High-pressure protective balloon deployment between the driver and the steering wheel is now installed in many new cars as a standard safety feature; in almost all luxury cars it is available for both the driver and front-seat passenger. On collision, a closed and strategically positioned balloon is rapidly inflated by a pressurised gas canister. The inflated balloon is then automatically interposed between the driver and the windscreen or the steering wheel. Thus deceleration impact is buffered. Recently, in the USA 34 child-deaths have been recorded as attributable to craniocervical injuries contributed to by air bags, mainly front seat. This has led to awareness of introducing "smart" (body-size selective) air bags. The combination of inertia lap-and-shoulder belts, head rests, air-bag systems and safer designs of consoles, instrument panels and laminated windscreens have gone a long way towards minimising physical injuries in RTAs.

6 Fire Burns

Fire burns to the neck in isolation are rare. Usually, such burns cause injury to the region of the face, the chest as well as to the neck. A common source of such an injury is faulty cooking equipment used with impunity and carelessness. Electric cookers are the safest and the rare instances of local thermal burns are confined to the hands.

With gas cookers operated by a piped gas supply, the damage to the neck is usually superficial; the main damage being to the trunk caused by ignition of the inflammable clothes, to the head (due to ignition of hair) and to the face and trunk due to explosion. Stored butane gas cylinder-charged cookers can explode from faulty design, unsafe handling and leakage, producing fire burns to the face and neck. Fuel-fired (pressurised paraffin-charged) cookers, also known as stoves, are still popular in many developing countries and occasionally explode due to faulty design or misuse, with subsequent splashing of the fuel. In this situation, fuel and fire burns to the eyes are common in addition to burns to the neck and the chest. Many deaths occur due to lack of safety awareness; the situation is compounded by users wearing combustible and inflammable clothes while cooking on such equipment. Skin is burnt depending on the extent of exposure to fire and contact with fuel.

The skin of the neck in the ethnic African and the Asian patients (being more prone to keloid formation), can result in massive disfigurement. There is usually an abundance of fibrosis produced in the region of the neck following recovery from such burns.

Management of fuel burns includes protection and care of the eyes and respiratory passages. Eyes should be examined for corneal ulcerations, if necessary by fluorescein staining. If evidence of injury is present, then chloramphenicol drops and an eye pad should be applied until specialist treatment becomes available. Prevention of blinking lessens further damage to the cornea.

Skin burns are treated on merit. Partial thickness burns generally granulate well although; some scarring and disfigurement may persist. Treatment includes administration of tetanus toxoid, antibiotics and an antihistamine. Use of topical steroids is controversial. An open method of treatment is preferable.

Subdermal fibrosis can result in keloid formation in susceptible patients, and this is largely unpreventable.

Full thickness burns to the neck impose many functional and cosmetic problems on the patient. Treatment includes antitetanus vaccine, antibiotics and delayed primary split skin grafting.

If subcutaneous tissue and muscle are involved and have to be excised, then a vascularised musculocutaneous flap can be rotated to cover the skin defect.

Inhalation of fire fumes, smoke or steam can cause severe acute laryngeal oedema with acute inflammatory reaction and carbon deposits in the lungs,[16,17] pulmonary oedema and pneumonitis.

Inhalation pneumonitis should be suspected if respiratory discomfort, pleuritic pain or haemoptysis occur. This is soon converted to a bacterial pneumonitis. Antibiotics and controlled chest physiotherapy are essential. Occasionally severe reactionary bronchospasms can be produced from smoke or toxic fume inhalation.

If the superficial fire burns are extensive, then disseminated intravascular coagulation (DIC) can result, due to excessive activation of thromboplastin. Management is complex and is best carried out in an intensive care unit with careful control of haemostatic factors, in addition to resuscitation and appropriate local treatment of burns.

7 Scalds and Insect Bites

Accidental water scalds to the face and to the neck can occur when a boiling kettle falls. A common variety of water or steam scald to the neck is produced by car radiators when a driver inadvertently uncaps the radiator of an overheated car. A blast of steam and boiling water damage the face and the associated part of the neck. This is probably the commonest accidental variety of steam scald produced to the region of the neck in adult men. Treatment includes analgesia, topical anaesthesia, antibiotics and in selected circumstances, topical corticosteroids. Antitetanus protection is also necessary.

When an irritant substance such as a strong alkali or acid is thrown at the victim a chemical scald is produced. Usually the face is the intended target and the substance trickles down the neck to the chest. Skin burns, toxin absorption and inhalation of toxic fumes all contribute to the overall injury.

Residual acid or alkali can continue to cause further contact damage to the skin, therefore these should be washed off and the area adequately rinsed with water. Some noxious substances (e.g. fire extinguisher snow) have specific antidotes printed on the container, and if available, these should be used in conjunction with other treatments. Further treatment is provided as for partial or full thickness fire burns to skin.

Many cases are on record of attempted suicides or torture where oral ingestion of noxious agents has been associated with contact burns of the side of the face and the neck. Oral ingestion can produce serious injuries. Corrosives such as mineral or organic acids (hydrochloric acid, sulphuric acid, nitric acid, acetic acid, oxalic acid), strong alkalis (Lye, caustic soda, caustic potash, ammonia), phenol and cresol (present in household disinfectants) can cause severe injuries to the oropharynx, oesophagus and even to the trachea.[16,17]

Petrol bombs produce a mixture of injuries. Facial burns, trickling fuel burns and fuel inhalation damage are all produced with such injuries, with disastrous consequences. Fuel scalds relating to substandard gas and fuel cookers (stoves) have already been described earlier (see section 16).

Surface injuries to the neck can be caused by insect bites. Local manifestations are minor, but generalised reactions from such chemical poisons may be out of proportion to the skin surface area involved.

Hornet, wasp and bee stings to the neck can produce a severe allergic reaction, leading to acute laryngeal oedema and death.

Removal of the sting may help as well, if visible on the surface of the skin, before tissue oedema conceals it. Bees leave behind a sting that continues to pump the stored toxin into the human body. Recurrent stings are more dangerous in producing an anaphylactic reaction. Corticosteroids, adrenaline, intubation and tracheostomy may have to be considered.

8 Deceleration Injuries of the Neck

These are associated with high-performance car accidents and falls from heights. As the victim decelerates, the viscera continue to move forwards at the terminal velocity. This tears the blood vessels and visceral vascular pedicles from the points of attachment.

Road traffic accident (RTA) whiplash injuries to the cervical spine and to spinal cord and are discussed more fully elsewhere (see section 26). RTA deceleration injuries produce a whiplashing of the neck at numerous levels. As the vehicle comes to a sudden stop in an accident, the passenger's body continues to move forward. This deceleration is prevented by the activated inertia seat-belt that locks the shoulder strap and the lap belt. However, the restraining effects of the safety belt are confined to the trunk and to the pelvis. The neck continues to decelerate forwards in its upper part. Acute cervical flexion with stretching is thus transiently produced. This is followed by a reflex recoil which produces hyperextension like a whiplash[13-15] (see section 5.4).

Whiplashing of the neck can occur at various levels, depending on the posture of the victim and the force applied. When an impact occurs, the occupant of the car continues to decelerate forwards. This movement is suddenly restrained by the seat-belt and/or the air bag system. The body is held rigid by the belts but the neck continues to decelerate forward until the reflex recoil reciprocally brings it backwards like a whiplash. This force produces severe localised damage to the susceptible parts of the cervical spine and the cervical spinal cord (see section 26).

Deceleration and impact injuries can also produce a violent shearing of internal jugular vein (IJV). Such injuries are usually fatal and are associated with more obvious injuries elsewhere (brain, chest, abdomen). When a large vehicle runs over a person, the skin and the underlying tissue is pushed forward with the wheel and this tears the nutrient and musculocutaneous vessels.

Rare impaction injuries to the cervical spine in rear seat occupants of a car (see section 26) have been occasionally documented when the car somersaults (cf. diving impact injuries).

Ejection seat injuries to the neck can occur during an aviation emergency. The rocket-fired seat goes through the canopy producing an impact injury through the pilot's helmet.

9 Traction Injury of the Neck

Traction injury of the neck can occur with skeletal traction for displaced fractures of the cervical spine. Many structures can be injured in unguarded or inappropriately applied traction. Posterior inferior cerebellar artery ischaemia due to compression of the vertebral artery has been reported.[18] Zimmerman *et al.*[19] have stated that traction is more likely to injure the vertebral arteries than hyperextension or rotations.

Chiropractic manipulations of the neck for spondylosis, osteoarthrosis or torticollis and so on can produce vertebral artery thrombosis and cervical spine fractures. This is not very uncommon.[20,21]

Traction during transportation may similarly cause acute vertebral artery ischaemia or may produce complete cord transection in a patient who might have initially sustained only a partial lesion of the cord.[22] It is difficult to quantify such iatrogenic injuries and therefore no reliable statistics are available.

10 Vibration and Blast Injuries of the Neck

An example of vibration and blast neck injuries in civilian practice is the vibratory injury caused by a bullet passing in the vicinity of a sensitive structure, such as the carotid artery. The kinetic energy of the missile (bullet or shrapnel) can produce vibration-related damage to the underlying or nearby neurovascular structures, if these are in close proximity. The injury is related to shock-wave transmission of force from the projectile to the host tissue (see section 4.2.3) and may occur even without a breach of skin.

Extracorporeal blast injuries (bomb blast or gas explosion) are comparable to vibration injuries of bullets and such damage generally includes injuries to the lungs and to other hollow viscera.

Injured nerves may develop reactionary neuropraxia. A nearby artery may develop a pseudoaneurysm from weakening of the wall produced by vibratory forces. Similarly, if the vibratory damage has produced injury to two adjacent blood vessels then an arteriovenous fistula may be produced.

Arterial and venous thromboses can be caused by such vibration injuries, although this is very rare.

Extracorporeal shock waves passing near a sensitive part (air- or water-filled tissues) may produce closed intrinsic damage. Such injuries are more common in the abdomen (bowel) and in the chest (lungs) but can also occur elsewhere.

11 Iatrogenic Injuries

The popular description of a neck injury usually relates to an external trauma of the neck such as a stab wound or a gunshot injury. It is only in the past few years that the concept has expanded to include iatrogenic injuries from diagnostic or therapeutic procedures. Many of these, in the neck, now occur during interventional radiology.

Cervical myelography can produce cord transection or myelocele with resultant Brown–Séquard lesion. Spinal fusion for lesions of the cord, unstable fractures or severe osteoarthrosis can result in an inadvertent iatrogenic injury to the cord itself.

Carotid angiography may lead to an arterial dissection.[23] Therapeutic embolisations of the external carotid artery aneurysm may result in stroke or death from embolisation of gelfoam fragments into the internal carotid circuit. Transfemoral Seldinger's technique has now largely replaced direct carotid puncture angiography and this has reduced the incidence of dissections and pseudoaneurysms,[17,23] but even simple and carefully performed vertebral angiography can lead to transient occipital lobe dysfunction.[17,23,24]

Internal jugular vein cannulation[25,26] can cause venous laceration or sepsis.[26] Badly attempted infraclavicular subclavian venous cannulations may damage the thoracic duct on the left side or may cause lacerations of the innominate vein. Other early complications include haematoma, arterial punctures, brachial plexus injury, air and catheter-tip embolism.[26] Late complications include thrombophlebitis, infection, late air embolism, arteriovenous fistula and local compression by an expanding haematoma.[17]

Exploration of the neck by a less experienced surgeon may lead to neurovascular damage in the subclavian triangle. It is periodically mentioned in the international literature that occasionally the roots of the brachial plexus may be accidentally transected by cautery or divided in mistake for the scalenus anterior muscle! Unfortunately, this is not all that rare where thoracic outlet decompressions are performed by less-experienced surgeons!

Carotid body tumours and thrombosed aneurysms have been explored with the mistaken preoperative diagnoses of cervical glandular tuberculosis or Hodgkin's disease, with disastrous results.

Operations on the cervical oesophagus may cause damage to the carotid artery, recurrent laryngeal nerve or the vagus nerve.

Blind plunging of a haemostat during thyroid surgery (if a vascular-pedicle ligature slips), may damage major vessels of the neck.

Laryngotracheal injuries can be caused during anterior mediastinal surgery such as for thymoma or for teratoma.[16]

Endoscopy may perforate the cervical oesophagus in a poorly prepared patient, producing cervicothoracic mediastinitis. Similarly, laryngoscopy, endotracheal intubation, translaryngoscopic biopsies, and so on are all associated with regional visceral injuries.

Following irradiation of the neck, skin burns, venous thromboses and neuritis are rare, but well-documented instances of iatrogenic neck injuries.[27]

We should also include in this group transport injuries of the neck. Here an initial neck injury may be made worse during unguarded transport in a trolley or in an ambulance (e.g. partial transection of the cord may become complete during lifting and transport of a patient without a cervical collar or a splint[28]). Chiropractic manipulations of the neck by untrained personnel may disrupt the cervical spine, cause damage to the nerves or produce vertebral artery thrombosis, in addition to causing other injuries in the area.[21]

Hurriedly performed tracheostomy or cricothyroidostomy especially with poor assistance can result in injuries to larynx, oesophagus, thyroid and major vessels. Careless endotracheal intubation of a patient with severe cervical spondylosis during anaesthesia can produce fracture and dislocation of cervical spine. The list of such iatrogenic injuries is endless but the important thing to remember is that most of these are avoidable!

12 Incidence of Neck Injuries

The incidence of isolated neck injuries is extremely difficult to evaluate because these are very rare. When these do occur they are often fatal. Neck injuries usually occur with multiple or craniofacial injuries.

The criminal, occupational or accidental varieties of isolated neck injury have not significantly increased in recent years. However, the incidence of combined injuries of the neck and of the adjacent areas such as the head, face and the thorax appear to have increased in various specific circumstances. The vast improvement of resuscitation procedures in the past 10 years has meant that more patients with multiple injuries are saved and therefore the incidence of survivors of combined neck injuries has increased.

Criminal injuries of the neck appear to have followed a particular pattern. In the developed urban communities, road traffic accident (RTA) injuries to the neck, if these can be classed as "criminal" at all, surpass other criminal modes of injuries.

Concomitant neck injuries (neck injuries occurring with skull, trunk or limb injuries) have increased in incidence, particularly in Afro-Asian and Latin American countries. This increase in incidence can largely be related to the limited use of restraining seat-belts and to lack of public safety as far as car decorations and driving standards are concerned.

Road-accident-related neck injuries cause more damage to the driver than to the front seat passengers of the car.

Criminal assaults, resulting in neck injuries, occur mainly from stabbing. These also do not occur in the region of the neck in isolation, and usually involve craniofacial or associated thoracic injuries as well.

Unfortunately neck injuries caused by knives are almost as common as those caused by guns in urban areas of most countries. Internationally, knife injuries are more common than gunshot injuries, but gunshot injuries are more frequently fatal. In the rural and, in particular, in the agricultural parts of less well-developed countries, the incidence of RTA injuries to the neck is low. The incidence of knife-inflicted neck injuries is probably the same as that of gun-inflicted neck injuries in such geographical areas.

Occupational injuries of the neck, such as those affecting professional couriers, have been increasing in the recent past. Motorcycle couriers transporting documents at high speed around a city sustain neck and other injuries more often nowadays. Neck injuries may be trivial or fatal (caused by impaction, twisting or crushing fractures). Associated brachial plexus syndrome may also occur in such motorcyclists.

The incidence of neck injuries is higher in industrial labourers working in foundries and dealing with ironmongery as compared with other trades. Neck injuries relating to farming or to agricultural activities are now reduced in incidence, even in less well-developed countries.

By far the commonest non-criminal injuries to the neck occur as a result of accidental falls. Here too neck injuries do not occur in isolation, but are usually associated with head and/or trunk injuries.

13 Incidence of Vascular Injuries of the Neck

Vascular injuries are easily detected if shock, massive bleeding or an expanding haematoma are evident. However, in the early stages, these features may not be present and the injury may remain occult for a while. A high index of suspicion is required for proper management of neck injuries, especially when penetrating trauma has caused the injury. All palpable head and neck pulses should be examined and bilaterally compared. The possibility of unilateral partial vessel injury must be kept in mind when these pulses appear equal.[29]

Table 13.1 lists the statistics of vascular injuries recorded at the Ben Taub Hospital, Houston, Texas for one year.

Table 13.1 Annual vascular injuries at the Ben Taub Hospital, Houston, Texas (modified after Feliciano et al.[30])

Location	Arterial injury	Venous injury	Total
Neck	17	34	51 (12%)
Chest	40	24	64 (16%)
Abdomen	41	89	130 (32%)
Extremity	123	40	163 (40%)
Total	221 (54%)	187 (46%)	408 (100%)

Reproduced with permission from *Annals of Surgery* **199**: 717–724, 1984.

Carotid sheath trauma includes acute injuries to the common carotid artery (CCA), its principal branches, the external carotid artery (ECA) and the internal carotid artery (ICA). It also includes injuries to the internal jugular vein (IJV) and the vagus nerve. The majority of such injuries are caused by deep incisional wounds (puncture) or lacerating trauma from penetration of a foreign body, such as a knife or bullet. It is rare for the ICA to be injured in isolation. The CCA is more likely to be injured by a bullet or a knife. The ECA is the next most frequent. Its branches overhang the carotid bifurcation and can bleed profusely. When the ICA is found injured by a penetrating trauma, other vessels and related regional structures are almost always injured as well.

Major arterial neck injuries can involve the terminal innominate artery, the proximal subclavian artery and its branches (thyrocervical and costocervical trunks), the CCA, its bifurcation and major branches of the ECA. Vertebral arteries are also injured, although rarely, from penetrating trauma, chiropractic manipulations and iatrogenically.[31,32] Vascular injuries around the thoracic outlet region constitute 4% of all vascular injuries.

On relatively rare occasions, blunt injuries to the neck may result in acute thrombosis of the carotid artery, resulting in stroke or death. Such injuries (producing thrombosis) may also be caused by chiropractic manoeuvres (forced neck manipulations) and hyperextension such as in falls and in RTAs, resulting in intimal tears.[32,33]

Venous injuries include injuries of the IJV (rarely the innominate vein), but the external jugular vein and veins in the vicinity may also be injured.

14 General Features of Vascular Injuries

14.1 General Features of Arterial Injuries

Arterial injuries can produce dramatic haemorrhage and are difficult to control. However, on other occasions, even a puncture caused by a bullet can self-seal and will then produce delayed disorders. In the neck, acute thrombosis or secondary compression can all produce intracranial ischaemic lesions and the signs and symptoms of these disorders must be carefully noted. The delayed effects are slow to develop but are potentially dangerous. Carefully selected patients can be observed pending arteriography. But such an observation must necessarily be frequent, such as every 15 min or at the most every hour. If such a frequent and regular monitoring of penetrating trauma of the neck is not possible due to staff shortages or due to lack of resources, then there is little justification of expectant management and an operative management is mandatory.

An injury to the region of the carotid sheath may result in profuse haemorrhage, shock (hypovolaemic or neurogenic), expanding haematoma, surgical emphysema, dissection or thrombosis of the carotid artery. Arterial thrombosis may lead to ipsilateral stroke. The internal jugular vein (IJV) may become thrombosed from compression. An IJV thrombus may become detached, resulting in pulmonary embolism.

Although some patients present with continuing haemorrhage and require immediate exploration and haemostasis, the presentation to clinicians is occasionally subtle and innocuous. The diagnosis of carotid sheath injury may require a high index of suspicion on the part of the clinician and facilities for appropriate vascular investigations. As a delayed consequence of such vascular injuries, a haematoma may become organised and may cause local compressive disorders.

An aneurysm or a slow dissection may arise from the injured carotid artery. Adjacent vascular injuries may produce an arteriovenous (caroticojugular) fistula.

Injuries to the vagus nerve may result in its division, a state of vagal shock or neuroma formation.

In the next chapter, arterial injuries are discussed in the following format:

● *Carotid artery injuries*

Immediate effects	Delayed effects
Haemorrhage/shock	Haematoma
Haematoma	Aneurysm
Intimal flap/dissection	Dissection
Thrombosis	Arteriovenous fistula
Stroke	Extension thrombosis/embolism
Acute surgical emphysema	

● *Vertebral artery injuries*
● *Thyrocervical trunk injuries*

14.2 General Features of Venous Injuries

Although venous injuries are less dramatic, they are often more difficult to repair than the arterial injuries. The haemorrhage may continue slowly to form a large haematoma and then the landmarks are obliterated.

Most venous injuries can initially be controlled by local compression, but these require formal exploration for repair and it is equally important to see if other structures are similarly injured. The injuries of significance relate to trauma to the internal and to the external jugular veins.

Venous injuries are discussed in the next chapter in the following format:

● *External jugular vein injury*
● *Internal jugular vein injury*

15 Immediate Effects of Carotid Arterial Injuries

The effects of an acute injury to the carotid tree in the neck are dramatic and usually abrupt. Major lacerations can produce rapid exsanguination, hypovolaemic shock and death. In such situations it is more important to stop or at least to slow down the haemorrhage than to spend precious time on volume restoration alone. When the first priority (haemostasis) has been achieved (usually direct firm manual pressure with a gauze pad or cotton-wool may achieve it) then rapid volume restoration must be undertaken initially with a colloid infusion and then with blood. If more clinicians are available, then initial haemostasis and volume restoration can and should be provided synchronously.

A large peripheral vein should be cannulated with a large bore needle/cannula, blood should be drawn for cross-matching and a small quantity stored for other less urgent investigations. Crystalloid infusion usually precedes colloid infusion to check cannulation.

While plasma expanders are in use, blood should be arranged quickly. In desperate situations, uncross-matched O-negative blood should be infused, but the ready availability of polygeline, plasma, albumin, and so on have all but eradicated use of uncross-matched blood. Respiration must be adequately maintained. Oxygen, through a mask and then, if necessary, through an endotracheal tube should be provided. A central venous pressure line should be connected up quickly for central volume assessment and an indwelling urinary catheter implanted to measure periodic output once the bladder is fully drained.

Other less dramatic effects of the acute arterial injuries of the neck are also described in this chapter.

15.1 Carotid Arterial Haemorrhage/Shock

The commonest result of a penetrating arterial trauma is profuse haemorrhage, resulting in hypovolaemic shock.

Exsanguination must be rapidly diagnosed on clinical parameters and volume should be restored quickly. A synchronous management of airway, ventilation and blood loss should be the aim of treatment. Endotracheal intubation, positive pressure ventilation with 100%

oxygen and "super large-bore" venous access are the backbone of therapy. Medical antishock trousers (MAST) should be used to redistribute blood from the periphery to the central pool and O-type blood should be used rapidly in such emergencies. Usually a massive transfusion becomes necessary and with that, increasingly, problems of mass transfusion are now being seen, such as citrate intoxication, hypothermia, microaggregate disorders, hepatitis (now non-A, non-B type), disseminated intravascular coagulation (DIC) and acquired immunodeficiency syndrome (AIDS).

The vast majority of carotid arterial punctures or penetrating injuries are fatal. In survivors, the wound may deceptively appear to be much smaller and innocuous than the extent of the intrinsic damage. Arterial haemorrhage immediately results in expansion of the surrounding area with an increasing haematoma. However, the area being deficient in deep fascia, the haematoma spreads fairly easily in all directions and often becomes "incompressible". In the early stages of arterial bleeding, because the soft tissue cannot resist the onslaught of arterial bleeding, the haematoma continues to spread unchecked. A mechanical digital compression of the haematoma in an attempt to stop its expansion during active bleeding fails because the hydraulic force is dissipated in all directions. Since sustained circumferential compression cannot be applied to the neck, the haematoma virtually becomes "incompressible".

As the haematoma continues to expand, the surrounding soft tissue is blood-logged. Gradually the pressure increases in the elastic confines of this potential cavity. Where sandwiching muscles or attachment of the superficial fascia to perichondrium is encountered, further egress of blood is resisted, in turn slowing the arterial leakage down.

All penetrating arterial injuries of the neck should be explored even if the patient appears to be fairly well and stable. Very often, the illusion of well-being is short lived and the patient develops reactionary haemorrhage. Delayed secondary haemorrhage or a large aneurysm may develop as a consequence. Resuscitation requires arrest or some initial reduction of arterial bleeding and this is often achieved by a gentle direct compression of the wound with a soft pad or gauze and cotton-wool. Success of the treatment relies on generous access, with adequate proximal and distal vascular control. In the situation of carotid arterial injuries the patient may bleed to death if proximal and distal controls are not readily achieved, since evacuation of haematoma restarts severe bleeding. For this particular reason the patient should be prepared on the operating table in such a manner that access can be obtained proximally and distally whether this would imply opening the chest or approaching the base of the skull.

If the clinical diagnosis is an arterial injury then the following steps are recommended for its management, while resuscitation is in progress.

1 Unilateral direct gentle compression should be maintained until the patient's condition is stabilised with restoration of blood volume.

2 The patient's informed consent should be taken for surgery ("exploration and repair") and arrangements should be made for the patient to be transferred to the operating theatre.

3 Since the eventual anaesthesia necessarily requires an adequate care of the patient's ventilation, limited exploration in the emergency room or exploration under a local anaesthesia are not good practices. The patient should be anaesthetised formally with an implanted endotracheal tube.

4 While anaesthesia and the operating arrangements are being made, availability should also be checked for a carotid shunt, a synthetic graft, appropriate vascular surgical instruments (including a range of bulldog or vascular clamps) and a sufficient supply of cross-matched blood. If hypovolaemia warrants immediate volume restoration then colloidal substances or plasma should be infused.

5 In certain well-defined conditions the use of O-negative uncross-matched blood is also justified, but with the availability of inert colloidal expanders such as polygeline, the use of uncross-matched blood should be drastically reduced.

6 In the operating theatre, facilities should also be available for measurement of the stump pressure of the carotid artery. Intra-operative angiography is not essential but may be helpful in selected cases. It can save valuable time.

7 When bleeding is very active, the approach should be rapid salvage. Initial control should be made of the bleeding with direct manual compression followed by an oblique incision over the anterior edge of sternomastoid. In the lower part of the neck, the common carotid artery (CCA) is isolated, looped with a sling for traction to produce haemostasis and preparations are made to cross-clamp the artery with a bulldog clamp at the right time. Similarly, the distal part of the CCA is similarly looped with a sling and prepared for clamping. Under such haemostatic control the wound is properly explored and the artery is inspected. If a part of the artery is neatly incised (stab wound), a suitable side-clamp can occasionally be applied and the other bulldog clamps removed to allow some forward blood flow along the carotid to the bifurcation. The artery is then repaired using polypropylene (Prolene) 4/0 or 5/0 sutures. After repair, the internal carotid artery (ICA) is bulldog-clamped and the side-clamp is removed. Any microclots in the entrapped area are then washed down the external carotid artery (ECA) circuit. Finally, ICA clamp is also removed. If direct arterial repair (arteriorrhaphy) is likely to produce stenosis then a vein patch angioplasty should be performed (see Figs 15.1 and 15.2).

8 When the bleeding is much less severe or when a good haemostasis has been obtained with prolonged local pressure, after adequate volume restoration and arrangement of adequate quantity of blood, consideration should be given for both life salvage as well as function salvage. Prolonged cross-clamping of the CCA (or the ICA) may cause ischaemic impairment of the ipsilateral cerebral hemisphere, if the contralateral ICA is not dominant enough to supply the contralateral (injured) side as well. In such cases, carotid shunting should be considered to allow cerebral circulation for the duration of arterial repair. To determine the need for carotid shunting, retrograde pressure (stump pressure) of the ICA should be measured as described below. In young patients, when the vessel has been actively traumatised and has bled enough to require local compression for temporary haemostasis, there is usually no need for carotid shunting. Shunting is necessary[34] when:

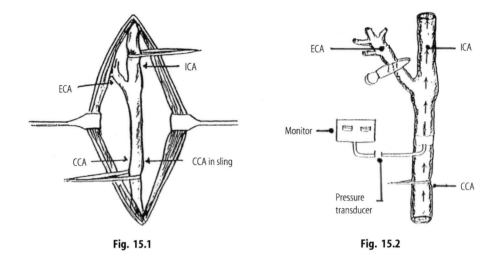

Fig. 15.1   **Fig. 15.2**

- neurological deficit is already present
- patient is elderly and suffers from an occlusive vascular disease of the neck vessels
- when repair of artery is likely to be prolonged.

In emergency situations especially with healthy young adults, the circle of Willis is competent with good cross-flow capacity allowing long periods of unilateral carotid cross-clamping with safety. However, on many occasions, general surgical trainees simply ligate both ends of the bleeding carotid artery. This is not a uniformly sound policy. The artery should be repaired properly. A hurried repair may lead to thrombosis or renewed bleeding. Carotid shunting is an easy and an excellent method of providing cerebral circulation allowing a proper unhurried repair of the damaged artery by arteriorrhaphy, angioplasty or grafting.

9 When the injury has involved an elderly patient, but after the crisis has been initially well controlled providing for somewhat better conditions, the ideal access is via an oblique incision along the anterior border of the sternomastoid which can be extended from the mastoid process to the jugular notch. Deep anterolateral lacerations of the neck should not be casually explored, without prior proximal and distal vascular control.

10 An essential policy should be to achieve a good proximal control initially, and this usually requires a separate proximal dissection in the lower part of the neck exposing the carotid sheath.

11 Once the CCA has been exposed it is cleared from the adjacent vein and a vascular (rubber) sling is used to encircle it in the form of a loop to act as a haemostatic control in times of crisis. The long sling is attached to an artery forceps that can be weighted down with a sponge-holding forceps to stop any ooze (Fig. 15.3).

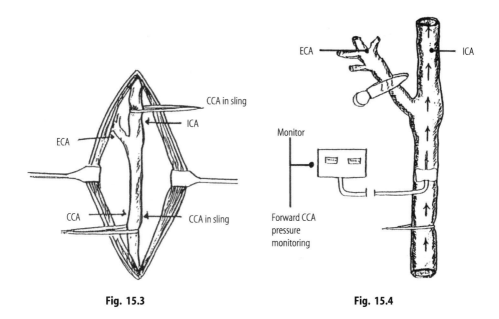

Fig. 15.3   Fig. 15.4

The retrograde flow returning from both the external as well as internal carotid arteries is such that the bleeding usually continues on, despite bulldog clamping or sling control (with manual compression) of the proximal CCA.

12 Therefore, a similar dissection must be made in the upper part of the neck anterior to the sternomastoid, in the described line and the carotid bifurcation is exposed. With adequate dissection of the artery from the vein, the carotid bifurcation is encircled and looped with a vascular sling. The bifurcation is then dissected and both the ECA and ICA are separately looped with slings. The ECA can alternatively be kept fully cross-clamped with a bulldog clamp or with a snugger without jeopardy during subsequent dissection.

13 At this point, the stump pressure of the ICA must be measured. The proximal CCA is cannulated with a small butterfly needle (21 G) that is attached to a pressure transducer (Fig. 15.4). The back flow of the blood in the tube of the butterfly needle measures the CCA forward pressure (e.g. the systolic arterial pressure of the CCA = 150 mmHg). The CCA proximal to the butterfly needle is clamped with a bulldog clamp. With the halt of the forward arterial flow, the artery distally reduces in diameter but is not devoid of blood. The blood within the lumen of the CCA at this stage represents the blood returning retrograde down the ICA into the CCA. This retrograde flow of blood has originated from the contralateral ICA via the functioning circle of the Willis (Fig. 15.5). The pressure within this "stump" of ICA and the CCA is now measured (e.g. stump pressure = 50 mmHg). The stump pressure represents the contralateral blood flow that has crossed over, after supplying both sides of the cerebral hemisphere (cross-cerebral blood flow). If this stump pressure is one-third or more of the principal forward pressure of the CCA (50/150 = 1/3) then it is deemed that the contralateral cross-over (cross-cerebral) blood circulation is adequate to maintain viability of both sides of the brain.

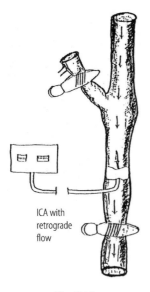

ICA with
retrograde
flow

Fig. 15.5

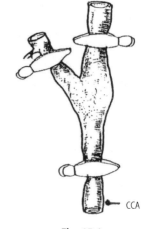

CCA

Fig. 15.6

With this knowledge, the surgeon is confident of not provoking a stroke by prolonged clamping of the CCA. First, intravenous heparin (5000 units) is injected peripherally and a minute later the CCA is cross-clamped as proximally as possible, to allow sufficient room. The ICA and the ECA are then clamped at their origins, separately (Fig. 15.6).

14 Following this vascular control, the actual wound is then explored.

15 The extent is assessed. Edges are debrided. Loose necrotic muscles are removed and the area of the arterial puncture or laceration is then fully exposed. If the artery is penetrated cleanly, producing an incision of the wall, then a simple primary closure (arteriorrhaphy) can suffice, using a non-absorbable smooth suture such as polypropylene (Prolene 5/0 for ICA and the ECA and 4/0 for the CCA) on an atraumatic needle. The incisions of the artery are repaired carefully, taking the entire wall in a manner that no kinking or stenosis should result. If the stump pressure is less than one-third of the CCA, forward pressure then cross-clamping of the CCA cannot be done for more than 3–4 min. In this situation, the ICA should be shunted (Brenner's shunt, Javid's shunt, etc.). The ICA and the proximal CCA are first looped with tapes and a tough plastic tube (snugger) is threaded to occlude their lumen. Peripheral intravenous heparin (5000 units) is infused and a minute later the ICA distally and the CCA proximally are cross-clamped with straight bulldog clamps. A small arteriotomy is quickly made on the ICA and the distal end of a carotid shunt is inserted. The clamp on the ICA is released and the tip of the shunt is advanced further quickly. The looped tape is now tightened with the plastic tube (snugger) and the position is secured with an artery forceps. A similar arteriotomy is made on the CCA, the clamp is released and the proximal tip of the shunt is advanced retrogradely. The loop is tightened. The shunting procedure under expert hands takes less than 3 min. If a Javid's shunt is used then Javid's shunt arterial clamps can be used to haemostatically compress the artery. With a carotid shunt in place perfusing the brain

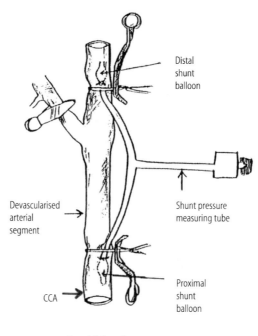

Carotid shunting

Fig. 15.7

hemisphere, further surgery can take place relatively more safely (Fig. 15.7). For every 30 min of shunting, the author recommends use of 2500 units of intravenous heparin.

16 If the injury to the carotid artery is so extensive as not to allow a direct primary repair of the lateral wall (lateral arteriorrhaphy), then vein patch angioplasty, vein interposition grafting (for ICA) or synthetic carotid bypass grafting (Figs 15.8 and 15.9) must be done. In exceptional circumstances, with mobilisation of carotid artery (with ligation of branches of ECA), sufficient length is gained to allow an end-to-end carotid anastomosis. In even rarer cases, an extra-anatomic bypass graft can vascularise the distal carotid artery (and the ICA). A common source of the extra-anatomic blood supply is from the subclavian artery. With zone I neck injuries, if the CCA is injured in its intrathoracic course and where a median sternotomy is indicated, such an extra-anatomic source of perfusion can be the ascending aorta. Although, statistically speaking, simple ligation of the CCA or the ICA for uncontrolled bleeding is the commonest treatment offered by general surgeons who are the first team to arrive on the scene, where vascular surgical expertise is available carotid ligation must never be practised. Lateral repair, onlay vein patch angioplasty, end-to-end arteriorrhaphy and synthetic grafting should be performed in this order of preference. A readily available graft is present in the form of external carotid artery that can be sacrificed for this purpose. If the diameter of the external carotid artery is much smaller, then it could be used either in the form of a circular patch or as a long onlay patch anastomosed to the freshened edges of the available wall of the native CCA. For a great majority of cases, if one arterial wall has been extensively

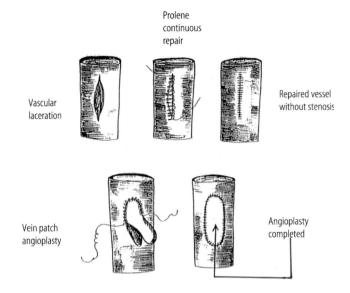

Prolene
continuous
repair

Vascular
laceration

Repaired vessel
without stenosis

Vein patch
angioplasty

Angioplasty
completed

Fig. 15.8

damaged then after adequate trimming of the injured area until healthy portions of the wall are in evidence, a vein patch may allow unstenosed restoration of the carotid flow. When even this is not possible, then the artery must be bypassed in its damaged segment, using an appropriately sized conduit (Fig. 15.9). The diameter of the long saphenous vein (LSV) is much smaller than the diameter of the common carotid artery but the LSV often matches the diameter of the internal carotid artery. Therefore when length deficit is present in the CCA requiring a conduit, then a synthetic graft must be used. Such grafts are used to restore continuity of the CCA, but usually not of the ICA. The author recommends the use of the ECA for restoration of the ICA continuity if only the ICA is damaged. But if both the ICA and the ECA are damaged then LSV should be used for the restoration of the ICA alone. Once the artery has been repaired, patched or bypass grafted, then due consideration must be given to preventing cerebral embolisation of any intrinsic thrombi.

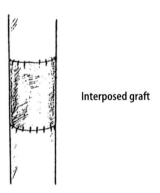

Interposed graft

Fig. 15.9

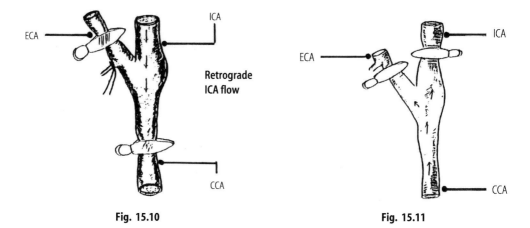

Fig. 15.10   **Fig. 15.11**

17 Flushing of the area before final sutures have been applied with heparinised saline ensures removal of debris and air. The isolated CCA is filled with saline and once debris and clots have been completely evacuated, the internal carotid artery clamp is released. This allows a retrograde filling of the CCA pushing down any thrombi that have been accumulating in the distal segment of the ICA (Fig. 15.10). The ICA is then once again clamped; immediately the CCA bulldog clamp is released. The blood is, at this stage, unable to go anywhere because both branches of the bifurcation are clamped (Fig. 15.11). The ECA bulldog clamp is removed next, discharging any leftover microemboli or air pockets into the ECA circuit (Fig. 15.12). Finally, the ICA bulldog clamp is also removed allowing normal antegrade circulation (Fig. 15.13). Once the repair has been satisfactorily performed and the area has been inspected for security of anastomosis, then the remainder of the area around the carotid sheath is carefully inspected again. On-table post-operative arteriography is very useful to confirm patency and any stenoses. If no ooze appears to be present in the surrounding area, then the wound can be closed without a drain.

18 If there is any doubt about the state of haemostasis in the perivascular area, then a small smooth suction drain is inserted, anchored and exteriorised into a sealed vacuum

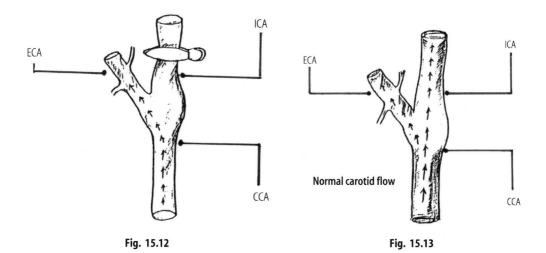

Fig. 15.12   **Fig. 15.13**

charged container via a separate stab. Trauma exogenously introduces microorganisms, in particular, Gram positive cocci, which join the endogenous pool of bacterial flora (which become pathologically active at the site of the injury and repair). Appropriate antibiotics must be given preoperatively, peroperatively and postoperatively. A suitable parenteral variety of cephalosporin should be given early in conjunction with a penicillin to cover the spectrum of such common microorganisms. If the wound is contaminated then antitetanus prophylaxis should be given as well.

19 Although primary haemostasis may be reassuring, at least two units of blood should remain available in the postoperative phase to tide the patient over, should there be any reactionary bleeding. The patient should be nursed in an intensive care unit where particular emphasis is given to maintaining adequate blood pressure. No anticoagulation is usually required postoperatively, but antibiotics should be continued for 5 days.

15.2 Acute Carotid Arterial Haematoma

The expanding haematoma offers a certain degree of resistance to the feeding artery when the limits of the deep layer of superficial fascia are reached, such as to the attachments with fibrochondral tissues. Because the superficial tissue is fairly elastic in the neck, the haematoma keeps expanding and the intra-cavity pressure keeps increasing. This increasing resistance slows down the continuing arterial bleeding. It needs to be emphasised that larger lacerations to carotid artery can produce exsanguinating haemorrhage to the point of death, therefore presence of arterial haematoma usually implies a small puncture wound, a small disruption or a fine pointed stab injury to the artery (Fig. 15.14).

This haematoma is usually pulsatile and the initial pulsatility can be reduced by a proximal compression of the carotid artery, at least in the early stages. When the haematoma has become large, the elastic recoil of the stretched tissue during diastole exerts a hydraulic compression force on the bleeding arterial point reducing the force of bleeding. When a larger puncture is present, the force of the arterial blood is so high that such compressive forces are unable to stop the arterial bleeding.

Arterial laceration   Arterial haematoma

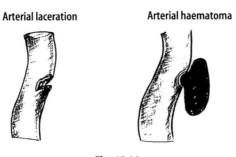

Fig. 15.14

A small initial haematoma is not necessarily representative of a "trivial" carotid injury, since there can eventually be a major blood loss from the initial puncture when arterial spasm resolves. No carotid arterial bleeding must therefore ever be regarded as trivial!

The management of a carotid arterial haematoma, following a recent injury, is the same as that previously described for arterial haemorrhage (see section 15.1). The main difference is that if the condition of the patient is fairly stable, then, prior to surgical exploration, appropriate investigations such as arteriography may allow a better definition of the extent of the injury. This must be balanced against the risks of sudden acute bleeding which could be difficult to manage on the X-ray table. Therefore, arteriography in such a situation can only be justified as an operative procedure – on the operating table!

A chest X-ray, estimation of haemoglobin and haematocrit concentration and proper cross-matching of appropriate quantity of blood should be performed. The haematoma must be surgically evacuated during an exploration and the arterial injury properly repaired. It should not be aspirated by a needle. To do this, the proximal part of the CCA and the carotid artery distal to the site of haematoma should be accessed by appropriate incisions and the appropriate segments of the artery slung with loops of rubber slings or tapes for haemostatic control (see section 15.1), should this become urgently necessary.

Once the proximal (CCA) and the distal carotid arteries (ICA and ECA) have been secured by vascular slings, then stump pressure of the carotid artery should be taken (if facilities permit). If the facilities for stump pressure measurement are not available then the carotid artery should be shunted under vascular control. Only then should the haematoma be dealt with. If active bleeding is in progress then there is no time to shunt and straightforward cross-clamping of the vessel proximal and distal to the site of bleeding must be carried out urgently. The wound is evacuated of haematoma, thoroughly explored and the extent of the arterial damage inspected and reconstructed by repair, patch or graft.

Smaller branches of the ECA are ligated and if needed, the main stem ECA can be fully ligated as well. The arterial injury is inspected, repaired under proximal and distal bulldog clamp control. It is mandatory to assess properly and fully the involvement of other structures/viscera as well.

15.3 Acute Dissection of the Carotid Artery

Acute dissection of the carotid artery can occur following a blunt injury to the neck when an initial bruising on the surface of the artery is followed by gradual weakening and then a dehiscence of the inner walls, leaving the tough adventia intact. Dissection can also follow a penetrating injury of the carotid artery where only part of a wall has been damaged. It can also be produced as a result of vibration or thermal trauma when intrinsic damage occurs to the walls of the artery by a bullet passing in the vicinity producing intense shockwaves. In such situations, the outer adventia is not damaged by the physical force of the bullet. It has also been seen after deceleration injuries of the neck in RTAs or similar accidents when mechanical shearing forces stretch the soft structures of the neck and produce disruption of part of the walls of the artery.[34]

In a typical arterial dissection, the tunica intima is breached and the cleavage is forcibly pulled apart by the entry of high pressure blood. A dissection (split) arises between the adjoining deeper layers of arterial wall and the high pressure of blood-flow tracks in the sandwiched parts, extending both longitudinally up and down the artery and transversely across the circumference, reducing the diameter of the arterial lumen (Figs 15.15 and 15.16).

Acute dissection can result from extrinsic injuries, but has nowadays become increasingly more common with interventional vascular radiology. Following a balloon angioplasty the disruption of atheroma may be associated with intimal injury resulting in an acute dissection. This can also occur as a result of guide-wire injuries to the intima and to the media of the carotid artery during selective catheterisation of the carotid tree by Seldinger's transfemoral angiography.

Once acute dissection has occurred, its extension along the longitudinal and the transverse axes of the artery occur rather quickly into the extracranial or even into the intracranial vasculature. The dissection may be incomplete, at least to start with, but eventually resulting

Longitudinal dissection

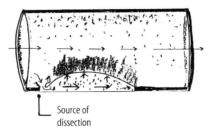

Source of
dissection

Fig. 15.15

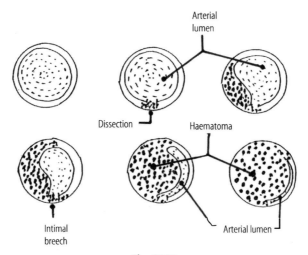

Fig. 15.16

in complete mechanical obstruction, producing cerebral ischaemia. Spontaneous atraumatic aortic dissections have been known to occur in elderly hypertensive patients, with plaque separation but this is very rare in the carotid tree. Autopsies of unexplained deaths consistently reveal a small number of aortic dissections in the elderly hypertensive patients.

A complete dissection produces a total or near total obstruction of the carotid artery resulting in acute cerebral ischaemia and stroke or death. A proper assessment must be made prior to haphazard or unplanned surgical exploration of the area.

If acute dissection has resulted in acute thrombosis, stroke and irreversible damage to the ipsilateral cerebral hemisphere then any surgical procedures to salvage the fully infarcted cerebral hemisphere are obviously illogical. The only place of surgery in such events is salvage of the unaffected parts of the intracranial contents. Such a salvage is therefore more preventive than therapeutic in value. Accordingly, this must be planned properly.

Dissection can occur retrogradely towards the aortic arch or antegradely to the cranial cavity, therefore relevant investigations showing the location and the extent of the dissection must precede definitive treatment. Preferably, conventional cineangiography or digital subtraction angiography (DSA) should be performed preoperatively. Duplex (and colour doppler) ultrasound study or oculoplethysmography (OPG) are not very helpful for this condition.[35]

Once the nature of the lesion has been fully assessed then formal exploration of the site of the dissection must be undertaken with a view to correcting the lesion. This can be done by closing off the area of the dissection by anchoring the intima and preventing re-entry of the blood (Fig. 15.17) or by end-to-end bypass grafting between the unaffected segments of the carotid artery (Fig. 15.18).

In this regard the ECA is expendable, and if it is found to be normal it can be used as a graft for the ICA. Apart from this readily available arterial graft, the best grafts for such a purpose are the long saphenous or the cephalic veins if no size difference exists. If mismatch of the size

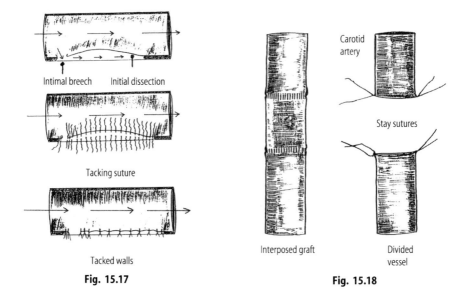

Intimal breech   Initial dissection

Tacking suture

Tacked walls

Fig. 15.17

Carotid artery

Stay sutures

Interposed graft   Divided vessel

Fig. 15.18

occurs then a synthetic Dacron graft should be used (Fig. 15.18). Grafting or angioplasty is followed by a full course of antibiotics, initial anticoagulation and subsequent indefinite antiplatelet therapy to prevent further local thrombosis and subsequent platelet embolisation.

15.4 Acute Stroke or Acute Transient Ischaemic Attacks

Following a carotid injury it is not unusual to find a minor degree of thrombosis developing locally and then embolising into the ipsilateral cerebral hemisphere. Such microthrombi are usually fragmented by the dynamic circulation or are fibrinolysed spontaneously.[36] Experimental evidence and considerable supportive clinical findings suggest a significant degree of stereotypicity in the path of platelet embolisation. In other words, each subsequent shower of platelets from a site of carotid plaque or thrombus is likely to travel to the same arterial branches where the previous shower of platelet had embolised.[35] Therefore, even a seemingly minor or a vague transient ischaemic attack (TIA) after a unilateral carotid traumatic thrombosis cannot be treated lightly. Significant thrombosis occurs frequently with a blunt trauma as with a penetrating injury.

Thrombosis can also occur following iatrogenic injuries such as interventional radiology (angiography, angioplasty or therapeutic embolisation) using Seldinger's technique.[37]

In the carotid artery, a small thrombus can propagate by extension into the cranial or in the caudal direction. Cranial thrombus-embolisation may produce a stroke.

Acute thrombosis results in mechanical obstruction to the blood flow within the lumen of the artery. A stenosis produces haemodynamic disturbances. A thrombus may produce a near total or total obstruction to the forward flow. If the ipsilateral cerebral hemisphere is not vascularised by contralateral blood flow (via a patent and adequate circle of Willis) then ipsilateral cerebral infarction may result (Fig. 15.19).

The substrate of energy for normal brain functions is principally glucose. Although the brain is able to utilise other substrates such as pyruvate in critical circumstances, the functional substrate of choice is glucose. If glucose is presented to the brain cells anaerobically then, via the Embden–Myerhoff pathway, the anaerobic glucose is metabolised into pyruvate with release of 2 mol of adenosine triphosphate (ATP) per mol of glucose. However, if oxygen is supplied, then the mitochondrial system is brought into action by activating the tricarboxylic pathway which metabolises glucose oxidatively, releasing 36 mol of ATP per mol of glucose. Thus, it can be seen that the availability of oxygen is a major factor in the production of ATP or energy necessary for brain functions.

Both glucose (substrate) and oxygen (fuel) are supplied to the brain tissue via an intact dynamic circulation. If the circulation is disrupted by thrombosis then obviously neither sufficient glucose nor sufficient oxygen are allowed to enter the ipsilateral cerebral hemisphere. If the circle of Willis is inefficient and cross-over (cross-cerebral) blood supply is minimal to the cerebral hemisphere principally affected by carotid thrombosis, then it

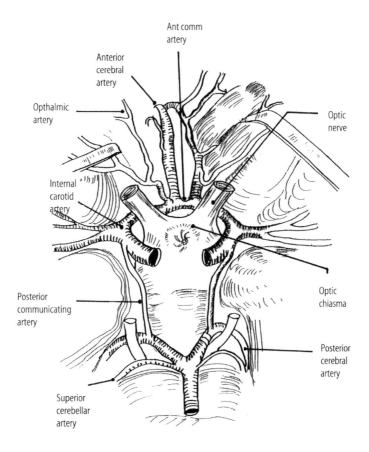

Fig. 15.19

would imply that the available oxygen is being used up at a greater speed than is supplied by the meagre blood supply of the opposite side. This will result in the glucose being supplied in the absence of oxygen. The substrate is thus metabolised anaerobically, resulting in accumulation of pyruvate and lactic acid byproducts with consequent development of acidosis and build up of carbon dioxide products.

The combination of hypoxia, acidosis and build up of metabolites, results in acute depression of brain functions. These make the initial effects of thrombosis-related cerebral ischaemia even worse.

The suspicion of acute stroke should arise when there is loss of consciousness following a blunt injury to the neck or following an interventional radiological procedure. The presence of cerebral ischaemic irritation can be detected by an electroencephalogram (EEG) and rapid sequencing contrast-enhanced computerised tomography (CT) scan of the brain or by magnetic resonance imaging (MRI).

The correct diagnosis can only be made from a combination of clinical assessment, non-invasive and invasive investigations.

An acute thrombosis of the carotid artery may exhibit absence of pulsations when the relevant side of the neck is examined but the transmitted pulsations from the pulsatile part of the carotid artery proximal to the site of the obstruction may be felt in the region of the thrombosis. There may or may not be a carotid bruit present.

Doppler can show cessation of forward flow of blood. Duplex and colour doppler can show stoppage of circulation at the site of thrombosis with proximal turbulence and distal retrograde flow. Conventional angiography or digital subtraction angiography can show the presence of acute thrombosis quite accurately.

If acute carotid thrombosis develops following an interventional radiological procedure or carotid angiography, then the treatment should be disobliteration of the artery, reversal of thrombosis and prevention of further stroke and TIAs. Thrombectomy or dissolution of the thrombus are the obvious methods of treatment available.[38]

Fresh thrombi may be susceptible to lysis with a fibrinolytic or a thrombolytic substance. In this context the roles of streptokinase and urokinase are well established. Tissue plasminogen activator is currently being used with good success as well.

Streptokinase is a product of Lancefield group C, beta-haemolytic streptococcal antigen, which has potentials of fibrinolysis and thrombolysis. Streptokinase is first bound to the circulating antibodies against the streptococcal antigen. The rest of the unbound streptokinase will result in fibrinolysis at the site of thrombosis by activating the plasminogen system. In other words, a certain part of the infused drug must be wasted on pre-existing streptococcal antibodies before fibrinolysis can start. In order for streptokinase to work efficiently a high initial loading dose is necessary to immunoparalyse the previously circulating streptococcal antibodies developed as a result of previous exposures to streptococcal infections.

Streptokinase acts by breaking off the intrinsic bonds of fibrin, resulting in release into the vasculature of fibrin-fibrinogen degradation products (FDPs) and loose unbound complexes of fibrinogen. This, in turn activates native plasminogen which results in lysis and unbonding of semisolid fibrin. Streptokinase tends to act on fresh thrombi and therefore such treatment should be given to patients who have recently developed a carotid thrombosis. Since detection of fresh thrombi and initiation of thrombolytic therapy both demand an urgency of action and availability of drug, the combination literally applies to those inpatients who have developed stroke in the premises of the hospital following iatrogenic injury to the carotid artery (such as by angiography).

Following the immunoparalysis, subsequent doses of streptokinase tend to fibrinolyse the available fibrin and produce lysis of the thrombus. Streptokinase should be given in the dose of 500 000 units as bolus, given by an infusion over a period of 30 min, followed by 200 000–300 000 units given intravenously every 4–6 hours.

Thrombolytic therapy should continue for 12–24 hours for pulmonary embolism, for up to 72 hours for venous thromboses and variably (up to 72 hours) for arterial thrombi including carotid thrombosis. After this, heparin therapy followed by a good combination of antiplatelet agents for preventive reasons should be considered.[39] The complications of streptokinase include streptococcal antigenic shock, renal compromise, protein-related reactions, pyrogenic disorders and so on. Urokinase is a much better thrombolytic preparation, manufactured from either foetal kidneys or from maternal urine. Cost-wise, urokinase is much more expensive. It has fewer side-effects and works on the same principles as streptokinase. The usual dose of urokinase is 2000 CTA units per pound, given intravenously in 10 min, followed by continuous intravenous infusion of 2000 units/lb/h.

Anistreplase, an acylated complex of human plasminogen and streptococcal streptokinase is a new product. The anisoyl group of this complex protects the catalytic centre of the complex, increasing the half life. The complex is taken up by the fresh thrombus and the anisoyl group is degraded within the thrombus. This activation converts the fibrin-bound plasminogen into plasmin which in turn, dissolves the clot. The drug is expensive and is administered as a bolus of 30 units as a slow intravenous injection over 3–4 min, within 6 hours of thrombosis.

Alteplase is a genetically engineered form of tissue plasminogen activator. It acts directly on the clot-bound fibrin and converts the clot plasminogen into plasmin. The risk of systemic bleeding is thus reduced. This is an expensive drug and is administered as a bolus of 100 mg intravenously over 3 hours.

Formal thrombectomy of the carotid artery should be done under the usual protocol which has been described for repairs of carotid artery (see section 15.1). Although the use of a shunt is unnecessary if a thrombus has already produced a 100% occlusion to start with.

Thrombectomy may be assisted with limited embolectomy performed by a catheter that should pull out a propagated thrombus from the extracranial part of the ICA beyond the reach of surgical exposure. The dangers of fractured plaques and loose fragments of clots embolising into the intracranial branches must be kept in mind. Embolectomy is controversial in this context. Frequent heparin/saline irrigation should also be done in between embolectomies. Intracranial embolectomy is controversial and the author does not recommend it. If it is at all performed then peroperative angiography must be done.

Following thrombectomy, the arteriotomy should be closed with Prolene 5/0 sutures without stenosis. Per-operative and postoperative anticoagulation should be maintained for a few days.

15.5 Acute Surgical Emphysema

Following injuries to the small branches of the ECA in the neck, there may continue to be a slow extravasation of blood that may track into various layers of the neck, depending on the track of the injury.

The carotid sheath contains a potential space which quickly fills up and then the extravasation leaks into the surrounding more superficial planes. As there is no deep fascia in this region of the neck, extravasation into the superficial layers is relatively easy. Blood spreads in all directions from the initial site of injury and may cross the midline to reach the opposite side.

Such extravasated blood conceals the landmarks of the neck and quickly produces doughiness and a "crepitus" which may be difficult to distinguish from emphysema related to tracheal or pleural injuries. A distinction must, however, be made in order to preserve the airway status of the patient and accordingly, tracheal injuries must be positively excluded in every case of vascular injury of the neck, where surgical emphysema is detected.

Usually the confined extravasated surgical emphysema is absorbed within a few days spontaneously, if no fresh bleeding occurs. Progressively increasing surgical emphysema implies a continuing slow haemorrhage and therefore the wound should be explored in order to achieve a better haemostasis.

At the time of the initial exploration, although major bleeding is more easily controlled, occasionally the smaller blood vessels undergo traumatic spasm resulting in temporary haemostasis. On recovery from anaesthetic, some of these blood vessels relax or vasodilate and resume the slow haemorrhage. If this reactionary haemorrhage is significant then, in addition to colloidal volume restoration, re-exploration should be done for better and direct haemostasis. If the emphysema is small, it will become absorbed soon, if it is large or increases then exploration will usually find the cause.

A major and relevant consideration is the prevention of infection in any accumulated haematoma and accordingly such patients should be given appropriate antibiotics (penicillin and cephalosporin). When re-exploration is undertaken to ligate the blood vessels, a vacuum drain should be inserted through a separate stab. The rate of infection is high and therefore prophylactic antibiotics should be liberally used in the presence of the drain, which should be removed after 24 hours.

Emphysema caused by leakage of air from respiratory passages (such as the trachea) as is seen after major trauma to the region or after major surgery involving laryngopharynx is discussed in the chapters dealing with these injuries separately (see sections 31 and 32).

16 Vertebral Artery Injuries

The vertebral artery is a deeply placed artery, protected within vertebral foramina but is liable to thromboses with acute and unguarded neck rotations,[20] chiropractic manipulations[20,21] and therapeutic traction[18,19](see section 9). Vertebral fractures and penetrating trauma can avulse it in the cervical part of its course, producing severe haemorrhage from both ends of the severed artery.

Vertebral arteries are seemingly well protected from external trauma as they pass through transverse foramina of the cervical vertebra, but they are vulnerable to neck rotations which can compress, stretch or twist these vessels.[20]

Dynamic angiography in patients and cadaveric blood flow studies[20] have shown that extreme contralateral head rotations with some degree of stretching of the neck can result in abrupt fall of the vertebral artery blood pressure to the point of total cessation of forward flow. If vertebral osteophytes from rheumatoid arthritis already exist, or if chronic malalignment from osteoarthrosis is present, then an arterial occlusion is more easily produced in vertebral arteries with extreme and repetitive neck rotations and chiropractic manipulations.[20]

Atlanto-axial subluxations produce two main neurological complications, compressive cervical neuropathy and vertebral artery insufficiency.

With penetrating trauma, because of its deep location, the vertebral artery is never injured in isolation and is usually associated with major trauma to related structures (roots of brachial plexus, trachea, oesophagus). Therefore, an overall regional assessment must be made as soon as temporary haemostasis (by extrinsic manual compression) is achieved. Ligation of both ends of severed artery is the usual method of definitive control offered, but where feasible, a direct repair or long saphenous vein interposition graft are better methods of treatment.

A penetrating injury involving the vertebral artery may also injure the cervical sympathetic chain, with resultant Horner's syndrome.

17 Thyrocervical Trunk Injuries

Subclavian triangle injuries caused by a stab or gunshot wound may disrupt major branches of this artery (Fig. 17.1). Arterial bleeding is deeply located and is always associated with additional injuries. The lower roots of the brachial plexus are in the vicinity and these are easily injured. Bleeding is usually profuse, but can be controlled temporarily by extrinsic compression. Simple proximal ligation is not sufficient because the vessels contributing to thyroid and scapular anastomoses will result in retrograde bleeding. Both ends of the thyrocervical trunk therefore, need to be ligated (Fig. 17.1). It is most unusual for this kind of an arterial injury to occur in isolation and therefore it is essential to assess the integrity of the adjacent structures as well.

On the left side, the thoracic duct can be injured easily, either with the initial injury or with the trauma of exploration. This results in a chylous ooze (see section 21.2). After surgical haemostasis, it is essential to explore the wound carefully to exclude such additional injuries.

The cervical sympathetic chain may become injured with an injury producing rupture of thyrocervical trunk. This may be the result of a penetrating trauma or may be caused by an unplanned and hurriedly performed surgery for haemostasis. Unilateral Horner's syndrome and a warm dry ipsilateral hand will then result.

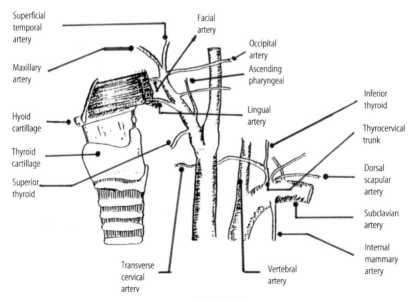

Fig. 17.1

18 External Jugular Vein Injury

Since the external jugular vein (EJV) is fairly superficial (Fig. 18.1) as compared to the structures of the carotid sheath, it is much more easily injured with various kinds of superficial trauma to the neck. A blunt injury may lacerate it but a much more likely disruption occurs due to an incisional or a puncture injury. A shotgun injury may avulse it altogether.

An injured external jugular vein (EJV) is easily compressible by external pressure and does not result in a major blood loss. It is usually associated with additional injuries such as injuries to the muscles and in particular to structure relating to thyroid gland (such as the

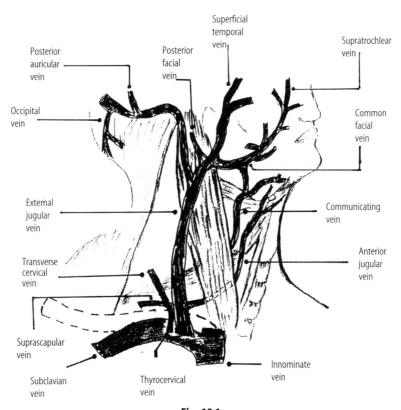

Fig. 18.1

blood vessels and the gland substance). Whatever the mechanism, the EJV may continue to bleed unless compression is applied and may build up into a large size haematoma.

When the EJV is totally disrupted, the bleeding may continue from both cut ends via numerous intercommunicating tributaries. The vein is easily controlled by packing or by extrinsic compression. It may stop bleeding spontaneously or may require ligation of both ends, after a formal exploration.

Since the EJV may not be injured in isolation, it would be entirely wrong to explore it under a local anaesthetic. The other more important structures should be explored carefully and major injuries excluded, before external jugular vein ligation alone should satisfy the surgeon.

Ligation of both EJVs will prevent adequate superficial venous drainage from the face and the scalp. At least one of the EJVs should be preserved, if possible.

19 Internal Jugular Vein Injuries

The internal jugular vein (IJV) is the major vein of the neck, transmitting ipsilateral intracranial blood towards the heart. It receives numerous tributaries, and most of these are fairly large vessels (Fig. 19.1). Because it is deeply situated, an injury to the IJV nearly always implies additional injuries to other important structures such as to the carotid artery, the vagus nerve and the viscera of the neck (the oesophagus, trachea, thyroid, larynx).

Iatrogenic injuries to the IJV are not that uncommon.[25] Cannulation may lacerate the IJV which may bleed considerably. Air embolism and catheter-tip embolism have also been reported.[26] Late complications include thrombophlebitis, infection, late air embolism, arteriovenous fistula (AVF), and haematoma-compression to adjacent structures.[26]

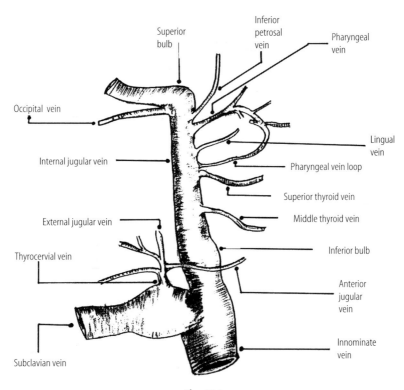

Fig. 19.1

In children, the IJV is frequently employed to draw blood samples. Tracheal injury has also been recorded during this procedure.[40]

Associated injuries cause additional problems. The resultant haemorrhage is profuse following an injury to the IJV and is very difficult to control. The best way of controlling such a massive haemorrhage is by local compression of the side of the neck, and quick and proper exploration with proximal and distal vascular control (both of the carotid artery as well as of the vein) is essential. With the ensuing haemorrhage from the IJV, gravity related embolisation may be produced. And this nearly always means propagation of a clot with or without an embolus into the right atrium, leading to pulmonary embolism with disastrous consequences.

Half-hearted attempts at haemostasis may result in suction of air into the empty part of the vein resulting in an air embolism. One of the major problems of IJV injury is the double injury related to the stabbing of the neck by a knife. Here, the IJV may be punctured and if the stabbing knife is allowed to stay in, the venous injury remains sealed with minimal blood leakage. With removal of the knife or the foreign body a renewal of major bleeding takes place, which is very difficult to control. Most of these penetrating injuries are through-and-through injuries of the vein and both venous walls need to be controlled for haemostasis. The main method of controlling this for a short period of time is to compress the area with a gauze applied locally and then to make arrangements for restoration of volume and exploration.

Ligation of one IJV can be compensated if the ipsilateral EJV is functional. Ligation of both IJVs will result in cerebral and facial oedema and considerable morbidity.

19.1 Surgical Options

19.1.1 Ligation

Ligation will produce haemostasis, but often results in acute cerebral oedema. It can also result in congestive disorders of the face and the side of the neck. If the repair looks difficult or if expertise is lacking, then ligation of both ends of the IJV should be performed with 3/0 silk or polypropylene. This is the commonest treatment offered, although a proper repair of the vein is by far the best method of treatment.

19.1.2 Repair

For repair to be properly carried out, appropriate clamps and suture materials (polypropylene) should be available. The venous wall is much more delicate than the arterial wall and therefore a greater dexterity is required for proper lateral repair of the venous injury.

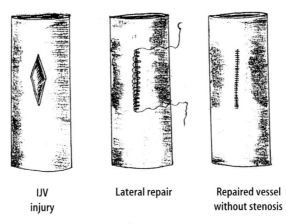

IJV   Lateral repair   Repaired vessel
injury   without stenosis

Fig. 19.2

With simple a haemostatic repair, a minor degree of stenosis may result with no appreciable cerebral oedema, therefore a quick lateral repair (using 5/0 or 6/0 Prolene sutures) should be the most practical solution (Fig. 19.2). There is usually a small ooze from the needle puncture sites. A gentle compression after repair will eventually control it.

Since the drainage of the head and neck can easily follow an alternative route if stenosis is produced (as a result of lateral repair of the vein), no major hardship arises as far as intracranial and arm venous returns are concerned, as long as only one side of the neck is involved.

When a large part of the venous wall has become damaged through injury or when trimming of the unhealthy parts of the vein results in the loss of more than one-third of the wall of the vein, then it is worthwhile undertaking a vein-patch angioplasty under vascular clamps. An adjacent vein such as the external jugular vein (EJV) is harvested and used from the same surgical access. Expulsion of trapped air and clots, just before the final sutures are tied, is essential. Any ooze from the site of repair can usually be controlled with compression with gauze for a couple of minutes. Venovenous angioplasty is much more difficult than a vein patch anastomosis to the side of an artery (Fig. 19.3).

19.1.3 Grafts

If the vein is so damaged that it cannot be repaired easily by direct venorrhaphy, then either a vein patch graft or a tubular graft (Fig. 19.4) should be used to restore continuity. Usually a venovenous patch suffices. Tubular graft thromboses easily after some time.

Whatever the form of treatment for the IJV injury, clot formation should be prevented following heamostasis and repair. If proper haemostasis has been achieved by proper repair of the IJV, then no appreciable bleeding takes place with proper anticoagulation. Anticoagulation should start per-operatively and should be provided with intravenous heparin. Heparinisation should continue until oral antiplatelet agents can exert their effects

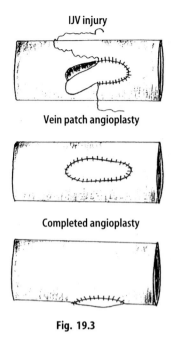

Fig. 19.3

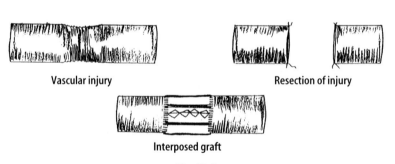

Fig. 19.4

in due course of time. Low molecular weight heparin is superior in this respect to the conventional heparin.

Since penetrating IJV injuries imply presence of injuries to other structures in the region as well, such as to the deep muscles, a very proper and meticulous surgical haemostasis is necessary, otherwise any form of anticoagulation will produce a haematoma.

Oral antiplatelet agents should be used for at least a few months so that the thrombogenecity of the new anastomosis (repair or graft) is reduced by endothelial proliferation and closure of the irritant surfaces by smooth endothelium.

If either an air embolism or pulmonary thrombo-embolism has been produced then the treatment will follow the guidelines for pulmonary embolism treatment.

20 Delayed Effects of Arterial Injuries

Not all arterial injuries are fully manifest on initial presentation clinically. Initial damage may be minor enough not to result in disruptive lacerations. Such examples are seen in shotgun injuries of the neck. One or two pellets may partially bruise the arterial wall. With the passage of time, the force of pulsatility may aggravate this damage and the wall may eventually rupture, producing haemorrhage, dissection or an aneurysm.

Fine puncture wounds of the artery are followed by intense vasospasm. This initially stops all bleeding. On casual exploration, all may appear well but when vasospasm resolves, renewed bleeding may take place.

Slow haemorrhage may be encased within rigid tissue and in due course of time perihaematoma fibrosis may wall it off altogether leading to the development of a false aneurysm.

Vibration or shock wave injuries may disrupt the arterial intima forming the basis of a slow dissection, but such dissections are more common with conventional angiography. During a catheter change for selective cannulation of carotid artery (especially the right common carotid artery), the *in situ* guide wire can erode the intima and this may not be apparent on subsequent contrast injections. The process of dissection usually starts immediately, but its clinical effects become manifest much later. I/V DSA study is much safer.

A bullet passing close to the carotid sheath may weaken the opposing walls of the CCA and the IJV. Over time, the arterial pulsations further weaken the arterial wall and the wall ruptures.[41] Following the initial injury caused by the bullet, there is usually a very intense vascular periadvential fibrosis produced and this anchors the two adjoining vessels. The disrupted CCA may thus leak into the IJV, creating a major arteriovenous fistula (AVF). Such an AVF can also be produced by sharp stabs lacerating both vessels.

20.1 Delayed Carotid Arterial Haematoma

With minor carotid injuries, such as fine punctures and stabs, the ensuing bleeding is minimal and the combined effects of arterial spasm, primary platelet plugging and increasing tissue resistance, tend to stop an obvious bleeding soon after the initial injury or at the time of surgical exploration. However, with reversal of spasm, such smaller vessels may spontaneously bleed, resulting in a haematoma formation.

The primary platelet plugs may not be strong enough to maintain haemostasis, with the result that with every systolic pulse, more pressure is exerted on the adherent platelet plugs. Eventually these may be disrupted and bleeding recommences.

Haemorrhage is initially confined to a small perivascular compartment. The surrounding pressure of the normal tissue, exerts considerable counter-pressure on the perivascular haematoma, limiting its expansion.

Sometimes, a few days after the trauma to the neck a haematoma adjacent to an artery may secondarily transmit arterial pulsations. Such arterial pulsations do not necessarily imply pulsatility within the haematoma unless a functional communication exists between the haematoma and the lumen of the injured artery (the pulsations may be "transmitted" and not "true"). The pulsating haematoma and surrounding tissue pressure work in opposition. A stage is reached when interstitial tissue resistance develops just enough reciprocal pressure to match the pressure of the progressing haematoma. When this equilibrium has been reached, the haematoma does not increase any further in size. At this stage the pulsatile nature of the haematoma encourages the surrounding tissue to generate a chronic inflammatory reaction and the junctional tissue slowly, but progressively, acquires a wall, encapsulating the haematoma – a false aneurysm!

If the arterial puncture or laceration, has by this time, healed over then the haematoma remains in isolation from the parent artery and acts like an encapsulated mass. Although unconnected to the lumen of the artery at this stage, it may continue to transmit an arterial impulse (transmitted pulsations). The swelling cannot be reduced with proximal compression of the carotid artery. Such an encapsulated haematoma may become spontaneously lysed and absorbed in due course of time, but this is rare. Encapsulated haematomas generally become condensed and organised.

If the haematoma is of a large size then during local lateral compression of the surrounding host tissue it may acquire an additional blood supply from the regional arteries to its wall. Thus, the capsule of the haematoma having arisen from a particular artery may now develop live vascular pedicles from other arteries that had been uninvolved with the original injury. Enucleation of the chronic haematoma may then necessitate ligation or cautery of these additional vascular pedicles.

Alternatively, the processes of organisation may result in thickening of the haematoma contents. Fibrous strands may develop from the surrounding host tissue, partitioning the haematoma into a multiloculated cavity. Slowly, further thickening may be followed by progressive calcium and other mineral deposition leading to the well-recognized radio-opacity.

It is most unusual for neck haematomas to behave in this way, but rare late sequelae such as calcifications have been documented from time to time. An organised or calcified haematoma may then persist forever and cause local compressive phenomena. Calcification of a mass raises suspicion of glandular tuberculosis more often than other conditions in Afro-Asian countries.

Until full encapsulation of the haematoma occurs, the introduced microorganisms (mainly Gram positive) and the bacteraemia-related Gram negative organisms may colonise the haematoma and produce local sepsis with abscess formation. This was typical in the pre-antibiotic era, but is still reported in the literature from time to time.

Such an acquired chronic abscess remains localised until breached by an injury (iatrogenic or introduced foreign bodies such as a knife) or activated by immunocompromising conditions (malignancy, radiotherapy or steroid therapy). With the reduction of the barrier, the abscess discharges, usually to skin, but on rare occasions it may find an area of low resistance in the hollow viscera of the neck such as the pharynx or the oesophagus.

20.2 Aneurysm of the Carotid Artery

A post-traumatic false aneurysm is a haematoma that maintains its communication with the injured parent artery and secondarily develops, as a result of condensation of the surrounding part, an acquired solid false capsule.[42] An aneurysm may continue to have an intact and functional cavity into which the blood circulates in a turbulent fashion or may become loculated following organisation or calcification of intrinsic thrombi. The larger an aneurysm, the more fibrous septa and loculations it possesses. The haemodynamic cavity may appear very much smaller on angiography than what appears on surgical exploration. In other words the mass of the aneurysm is always much bigger than its haemodynamic capacity.[41]

If an aneurysm becomes totally thrombosed it ceases to be haemodynamically functional, but may continue to cause local compressive injury to the surrounding structures.[22,43] Such totally thrombosed aneurysms may lose their pulsatility or the transmitted pulsations from the proximal artery may be too feeble to palpate. When palpating such thrombosed aneurysms, the risk of discharging emboli distally should be kept in mind.[43]

The false capsule of the aneurysm is fairly tough to be able to withstand the onslaught of arterial pulsations. With passage of time the fibrous capsule of the aneurysm is converted into a solid calcified shell which retains the configurations of the aneurysm, like the wrappings of an Egyptian mummy. If the initial arterial haematoma becomes organised in a small confined space, then the resultant aneurysm continues to be bombarded by haemodynamic circulatory forces. A large aneurysm has a greater capacity and the arterial pressure is quickly dissipated all around, resulting in a considerable reduction of arterial pressure during the systolic phase of aneurysmal filling. However, in smaller aneurysms there is not much loss of pressure and these remain more pulsatile. A small aneurysm is usually more pulsatile than a chronic large aneurysm. Pulsatility also relates to the amount of elastic tissue and this is relatively greater in the periphery.

If the haematoma causes local compression of the adjacent internal jugular vein, then the haematoma may erode the wall of the vein and may eventually open into it. The artery is thus connected to the vein via the haematoma and an arteriovenous aneurysm is produced. This situation is somewhat different to a direct communication between an injured artery and an injured vein, where a direct arteriovenous fistula (AVF) is produced. The haemodynamics of an arteriovenous aneurysm and those of the AVF are considerably dissimilar.

Initially, the pseudoaneurysm does not have a clot, but over time it develops one due to dynamic turbulence within the intrinsic cavity of the aneurysm. On a susceptible nidus the turbulent blood sets up an initial platelet plug followed by an adherent clot. The clot then acts as a nidus that attracts more platelet plugs. The mass may propagate through the ostium. One of the main dangers of intrapseudoaneurysmal thrombosis, is the discharge of minute particles as emboli into the distal circulation.[41]

A carotid pseudoaneurysm is quite capable of discharging such emboli and in producing transient ischaemic attacks (TIAs), amaurosis fugax (Afx) or stroke. It is for this potential of emboli formation that an internal carotid aneurysm is seldom embolised iatrogenically, using gelfoam, ivalon sponge or coiled springs etc although in expert hands it is possible.

If the arterial wall is injured at more than one site, then multiple ostia may be formed but this is unusual.

When a single ostium is present, the major pulsatile force is transmitted via this ostium and the force is dissipated into the cavity. The force, having been thus reduced, a single moderate-sized ostium prevents the formation of additional minor ostia in the vicinity.

The ECA pseudoaneurysms can be easily obliterated by iatrogenic gelfoam embolisation procedures provided that due care is taken to prevent reflux and clot embolisation into the internal carotid artery circuit.

A pseudoaneurysm should be fully and properly investigated. An extracranial carotid pseudoaneurysm may already have discharged emboli into the ipsilateral cerebral hemisphere producing areas of cerebral infarction or cerebral ischaemia.

An assessment of cerebral neurology is essential, followed by specific diagnostic investigations such as transcranial doppler study, nuclear magnetic resonance (NMR) scans, magnetic resonance imaging (MRI) or CT scans.

The extracranial aneurysm can be quite satisfactorily assessed with a duplex scan (pulsed doppler with a real-time 'B' mode ultrasound) or through a colour doppler (Dopscan, Triplex) showing directional flow changes and related turbulence as well.[41,42] Such an ultrasound study may show the pattern of the turbulent flow within the aneurysm. It may also show any distal kinking or stenosis of the internal carotid artery.

A relevant, easy-to-perform cerebral investigation, however, is the contrast-enhanced computerised tomography (CT) scan. Rapid sequencing CT scans show pre-infarcted ischaemia reasonably well. Nuclear magnetic resonance imaging (NMR or MRI) may also show such a lesion with reasonable accuracy, non-invasively. The most sensitive and specific investigation however, is some form of invasive or semi-invasive arterial study such as the cineangiography or cut-film angiography using a rapid cassette changer. Digital subtraction angiography (DSA), because of its low invasiveness, has gained considerable popularity.

The best resolutions of images in the head and neck vascular study come from an intra-arterial DSA. This can be performed via a proximal cannulation of the common carotid artery of the affected side (through a Seldinger femoral approach) and by injecting a small dose of an appropriate dye (76% urografin) recording the flow of the dye along the carotid artery and into the aneurysm on the "cineloop" of the DSA computer. This will show various phases of aneurysmal activities and may outline the nature of the ostium accurately. DSA performed via an arterial route is superior in quality to the DSA performed via an intravenous route but arterial DSAs are more invasive. In high flow situations, such as the carotid artery, intravenous dye is diluted many times and the arterial phase is not outlined very clearly. An intra-arterial DSA gives a very good resolution.

The invasiveness of the DSA lies in an arterial puncture, catheterisation and thrombogenecity of the viscous and irritant dye. Its invasiveness can be substantially reduced by placing the catheter in the proximal aortic arch. The dye is then diluted and both sides of the neck can be simultaneously studied and documented. In good hands, using various computer programmes, the computer image of the arterial tree obtained via an intravenous route can be enhanced to improve the clarity of resolution. For most diagnosis purposes, such an intravenous DSA may suffice, but an intra-arterial DSA is unquestionably superior. Proximal carotid catheterisation is much more invasive than aortic arch DSA but gives superior information. If biplane views are documented then a single-hand injection will give high-quality pictures. The choice of selecting the method of performing DSA (intravenous injections of the dye, aortic arch injections, proximal carotid catheter injections) rests with the treating vascular surgeon and the Vascular Radiologist. The value of these tests relate to the surgeon's personal experience. Observer error is considerably reduced if the treating surgeon participates in the DSA study or performs it himself or herself.[41]

In the author's opinion, the catheter should be placed in the relevant carotid artery proximally and specific images recorded on the computer, following the first-hand injection using a small quantity of contrast. Following heparin flush, the catheter should be withdrawn to the proximal aortic arch and a further injection given using a slightly larger quantity of dye. Such an arch injection should show bilateral carotid and vertebral arteries. If needs be, further similar injections can be given in a lateral position. Postural manipulations are made to achieve the best imaging of the carotid bifurcation. Both the extracranial and intracranial courses of these vessels should be recorded. After the injection, but before the catheter removal, images are carefully examined. Further computer manipulation and image enhancement can take place later on, using various software. Heparin flush minimises clot embolisation and should be done routinely.

The most reliable investigation is conventional angiography of the carotid tree, despite its invasiveness. This is the yardstick of all of the investigations relating to the anatomy of the carotid tree. The advantages of the conventional carotid angiography are that the aneurysm is outlined quite accurately showing its haemodynamic behaviour and anatomical pattern, if cineangiography mode is utilised. Conventional cut-film (X-ray plate) angiography is more invasive than the arterial DSA, but is cheaper and more readily available. Video recording of the phases of hand injection during conventional angiography (video-angiography) produces an inferior resolution of images, but is very cheap and can be easily displayed in an ordinary operating theatre. In developing countries this is a very useful investigation tool.[41]

Cineangiography outlines the aneurysm very well, showing intrinsic turbulence and any clots. Carotid distal flow (which is more importantly, the major consideration), is outlined more clearly.

During arch aortography (cineanagiography or DSA) the ipsilateral carotid artery can be compressed by fingers placed on the neck. This can show the degree of retrograde cerebral flow from the contralateral side. If the study shows a good contralateral carotid flow via a competent circle of Willis anastomosis, then the patient may be physiologically competent to withstand the prolonged cross-clamping of the ipsilateral ICA for an aneurysmectomy, an aneurysmorrhaphy or a bypass graft of the affected segment. However, there may be occasions when such a retrograde flow demonstrated on the cross-flow technique is inadequate for optimum cerebral perfusion. Such cross-cerebral flow studies are difficult to perform and are not without their own dangers. Once again, this is an observer-related exercise and the vascular surgeon should build his or her own experience in this technique.

One should always rely on direct measurement of retrograde carotid flow, cerebral blood flow studies or an intra-operative electroencephalogram (EEG) to ascertain if cross-clamping without shunting is justifiable (see section 15.1). In the author's view, mere demonstration of this retrograde flow radiologically is not sufficient proof of adequate cross-cerebral blood supply. The author recommends that arterial stump pressure should be measured at the time of surgery and if it is found to be low (less than one-third of forward pressure) then a carotid shunt must be used immediately prior to cross-clamping (Fig. 15.7). Similarly if the intra-operative EEG of the temporarily cross-clamped carotid artery exhibits cerebral distress within 3 min, then shunting must be undertaken prior to further cross-clamping. Cerebral blood flow studies can similarly provide information as to whether the ipsilateral cerebral hemisphere can tolerate cross-clamping without a protective shunt. Once the angiography has been studied properly (and this includes assessment of the vascularisation of the capsule of the aneurysm as well), then a formal surgical treatment can be planned.

If the external carotid artery (ECA) is the only part of the artery bearing the aneurysm, then the ECA aneurysm can be iatrogenically embolised via Seldinger's approach. However, care should be taken to prevent leakage of gelfoam and so on into the bifurcation or into the ICA. This technique is also helpful in preoperatively reducing vascularity of a carotid body tumour.[44]

Iatrogenic embolisation entails cannulation of the femoral artery by Seldinger's method. The angiography catheter is advanced under image intensifier vision to the carotid artery from where the aneurysm has arisen. Intermittent dilute dye injections outline the location of the ostium. At this point a soft-tipped curved angio-guide wire is introduced into the catheter and is negotiated into the lumen of the false aneurysm via the ostium. It may necessitate changing catheter size to one of a smaller diameter. Once the aneurysmal cavity has been reached via the soft guide wire then a soft embolisation type catheter is threaded over the guide wire, and is then negotiated into the aneurysmal cavity itself.

Such an embolisation catheter is a double lumen tube which transmits the dye or the embolising material via the terminal end while the lateral ostia can irrigate the lumen of the aneurysm with heparin. A further modification is the presence of a proximal balloon to prevent reflux of the embolising substance into the proximal artery. An ordinary multipurpose catheter can also be used if a proper embolisation catheter is not available.

With such a technique the aneurysmal cavity is slowly injected with an embolising inert material such as ivalon sponge, gelfoam, beads, thrombin and so on. Once the size of the cavity has been filled to some extent with such inert substances, then a choice lies between continuing with the injections of such sponges or embolising with detachable spring coils. Gradually, spring coils, beads or sponges are stacked up in the aneurysmal cavity until it is sealed off completely. It is necessary to seal it off as closely to the ostium as possible to prevent a secondary aneurysm formation.

The carotid aneurysm, thus embolised can be obliterated, but the aneurysmal space and the coagulated solid aneurysm will persist, causing local compression to the adjacent structures, such as to the vagus nerve, upper elements of the brachial plexus, internal jugular vein and the viscera of the neck, depending on its size.

Embolisation of CCA and ICA aneurysms is not very popular because of the high risks of inadvertent distal cerebral embolisation. An occasional death has been recorded from such embolising procedures. The ECA aneurysm can be easily embolised iatrogenically but with due care.

The relevant surgical treatment is ligation of the aneurysmal ostium and repair of the lateral wall of the carotid artery to restore continuity without causing any stenosis. The false capsule of the aneurysm is excised for decompression.[43]

In situations where the ostium of the aneurysm is wide (greater than 33% of the diameter of the artery), then it is essential after aneurysmectomy to repair the arterial defect with a vein patch, obtained from an adjacent vein. Such an angioplasty will ensure that no iatrogenic stenosis of the carotid artery results following the procedure.

If the aneurysm is irregular, large and complex, making the vein patch angioplasty inappropriate, or if the aneurysm has secondarily injured the wall of the carotid artery in a manner that it can not be repair easily, then an aneurysmectomy is followed by interposition bypass graft, using a synthetic conduit (Vascutek, Goretex, Impra grafts).

The common carotid artery (CCA) diameter is larger than that of the long saphenous vein and to avoid a mismatch a synthetic "size-for-size" graft is therefore selected. Aneurysmectomy cannot be performed adequately, using a side biting clamp and therefore cross-clamps are necessary.[45]

If bypass grafting is performed or if vein patch angioplasty is to be done then the carotid artery should be bull-dog clamped and for this, stump pressure measurements must be taken as explained earlier (see section 15.1), and if indicated a bypass shunt must be positioned prior to formal prolonged clamping of the common carotid artery (Fig. 15.7).

20.3 Delayed Carotid Dissection

Arterial dissection following an injury is a slow and self-propagating process arising after an iatrogenic injury to the artery (produced by arterial catheterisation, therapeutic embolisation) or blunt injuries of the neck.

The tunica intima splits, allowing blood to track within the outer linings of the artery, as a sandwiched "haematoma". Such an injury can also be intrinsically produced by the vibratory forces generated by blast or by a bullet passing nearby, weakening and disrupting the deeper arterial wall. Surprisingly, such a dissection can be caused by seemingly trivial injuries where the patient does not appear to have sustained a manifest major arterial damage immediately following an injury (Fig. 20.1).

Understandably, most rifle wounds of the neck are fatal. In only a small proportion of such rifle bullet injuries are the thermal and vibratory trauma high enough to produce a local area of weakening or damage of the tunica intima intrinsically.[46] Whatever the cause, if the tunica intima is disrupted then the pulsatile flow of the high-pressure blood will erode through the walls of the artery, sandwiching itself lengthwise and breadthwise between the media and the adventia or between the intima and the media.

Longitudinal tracking of the dissection progresses headwards towards the cranial cavity and it is quite possible for it to enter intracranial cavity as well. As a late event, the dissection can progress retrogradely towards the arch of the aorta. As the longitudinal dissection continues, the dissected blood bulges the intact intima into the lumen of the artery producing a longitudinal mechanical intrinsic stenosis.

Transverse dissection will also result in annular stenosis of the carotid artery. It is commoner for a longitudinal rather than for a transverse dissection to occur in extrinsic arterial injuries (Fig. 20.2).

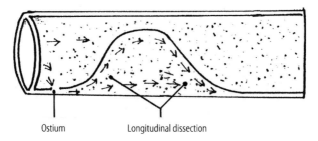

Ostium   Longitudinal dissection

Fig. 20.1

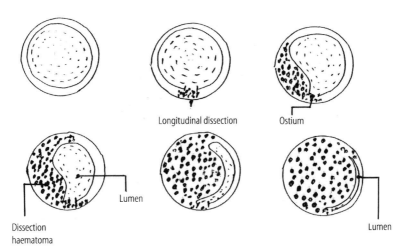

Longitudinal dissection   Ostium

Dissection
haematoma   Lumen   Lumen

Fig. 20.2

The pathological effects of such a delayed dissection following arterial trauma is thrombosis and local damage of the intima producing a nidus for platelet adhesions and headward embolisation of such platelet plugs.

Immediate pathological disorders include embolisation into extracranial circulation of platelet plugs and debris from detached arterial wall. Delayed disorders include atherosclerotic plaques and aneurysm formation.

Clinical features of dissection are variable and generally depend on the rapidity of onset of obstruction. When this occurs quickly and if the lesion is total (100%) of the CCA or the ICA, the resultant neurovascular shock can mimic haemorrhagic shock (falling blood pressure, rising pulse rate, cold clammy skin). These two "shocks" must be differentiated. In carotid dissections, as in aortic dissections, there is no actual hypovolaemia present as is indicated by a very high central venous pressure (CVP). Without this evaluation, there is a temptation to transfuse the patient with whole blood and such an injudicious transfusion in dissections will produce proximal cardiac overloading, adding to the myocardial strain. When the right carotid dissection descends towards the heart involving the innominate artery, the brachial blood pressure usually falls and may not be recordable in the right arm. A left-sided carotid dissection can descend to the aortic arch but seldom causes aortic occlusion.

Typical clinical features of acute carotid dissection also include features of cardiogenic shock, stroke or TIA. The patient may lose consciousness or may die.

Carotid dissection is very difficult to treat but prior to the treatment its full extent must be assessed properly. The only positive and useful investigation is cineangiography that is superior in outlining the dissection to digital subtraction angiography or to conventional angiography. Angiography must be performed carefully. It may show the dye ascending into the dissected area or indirectly producing a filling defect in the lumen. Magentic Resonance Arteriography (MRA) shows promise, as a new diagnostic tool.

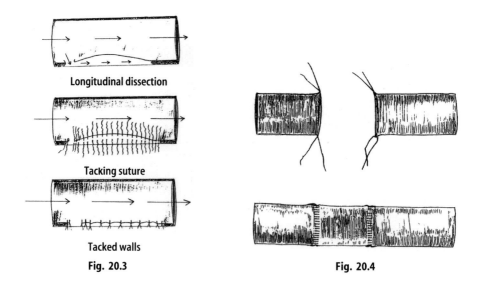

Longitudinal dissection

Tacking suture

Tacked walls

Fig. 20.3   **Fig. 20.4**

Once the extent of the dissection has been outlined and if it appears to be extracranial, then appropriate surgery is planned in the neck immediately. Such an angiography is best performed in the operating theatre using Seldinger's technique. If an operable lesion is found then general anaesthesia is commenced.

An intracranial extension is much more difficult to treat but can be managed by proper combined neurovascular resources (intracranial–extracranial bypass graft and ICA ligation).

Low extracranial carotid dissection occurring as a delayed complication of carotid arterial trauma, requires formal stump pressure measurements for bypass shunting followed by specific operations for treatment of dissection.

An easy, but less popular, operation is that of exposing the intima and tying or applying tacking sutures, fixing the intima with the adventia and entrapping the media within, thus obliterating the cavity. Such tacking sutures obliterate the dissected cavity and the source of dissection (Fig. 20.3).

However, despite such operations, the injury produced to the walls of the carotid artery may not recover fully and may not result in full dynamicity as far as carotid arterial circulation is concerned. A common policy therefore, is to excise the diseased segment and to replace it with a synthetic graft under a carotid bypass shunt, if indicated by a low stump pressure (Fig. 20.4).

20.4 Arteriovenous Fistula

In the neck region the main arteriovenous fistula (AVF) of interest is the caroticojugular fistula, caused usually by stabbing injuries or by gunshot injuries (Fig. 20.5),[43] but minor vessels can also produce fistulae.

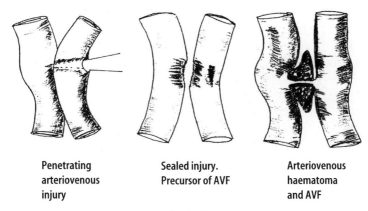

| Penetrating arteriovenous injury | Sealed injury. Precursor of AVF | Arteriovenous haematoma and AVF |

Fig. 20.5

Following a high velocity vibration injury to the neck (caused, for example, by the passage of a bullet nearby or an explosive blast in the vicinity), the walls of the artery and of the adjacent vein, may become acutely disrupted (resulting in profuse bleeding) or the vessel walls may simply be bruised and injured by the shockwaves. Such an injury is made progressively worse with the force of the arterial pulsations. First the muscles of the tunica media become inactive, atrophied and flat and give way to the blood that has already eroded the tunica intima. Then the adventia give way. Chronic inflammatory cells produce intense adhesion between the two vessels. The artery thus eventually leaks into the vein with very little extravasation into the perivascular tissue and an AVF is created (Fig. 20.5).

Another variety of the AVF is the development of a periarterial haematoma following blunt injury, gunshot wounds or stabs in the anterolateral aspects of the neck. The perivascular haematoma remains in continuity with the artery and therefore pulsates with the arterial pulse. The "pulsatile haematoma" gradually erodes through the adjacent wall of the intact vein and results in the formation of an "arteriovenous aneurysm". Thus the artery is connected to the vein by the haematoma (Fig. 20.6).

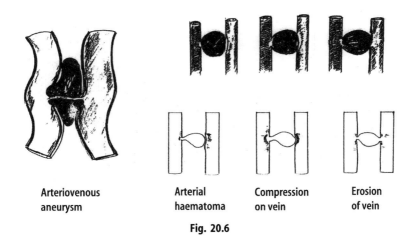

| Arteriovenous aneurysm | Arterial haematoma | Compression on vein | Erosion of vein |

Fig. 20.6

With the passage of time, the walls of the haematoma become organised and condensed, leaving behind a small track communicating the artery with the vein.

Thermal injuries, radiation injuries and mechanical trauma to the adjacent wall of the artery and the vein can also result in the development of a major AVF between the CCA and the internal jugular vein (IJV). Pathological neovascularisation or erosion of the local tissue by a fast enlarging malignant tumour in the region of the neck may produce an AVF, although this is rather rare. In general, the AVF produces both local effects as well as more pronounced generalised effects. Through a functioning ostium the haemodynamic pressure will self-propagate the lesion. The ostium may become thickly organised. At this point the AVF becomes permanent. The haemodynamics of the AVF are directly related to the size of the arterial pressure and to the size of the ostium. If the ostium is very narrow then the major flow of the arterial blood remains in the direction of the parent artery. A common carotid artery–internal jugular vein fistula (caroticojugular AVF), with a very narrow or small ostium, will transmit the bulk of the arterial blood into the carotid bifurcation. The blood loss via the fistula in such situations is small and the major direction of the fistulous transmission is towards the heart. Therefore, a small ostial fistula results in a near normality of the arterial blood-flow with only that part of the arterial blood leaking into the fistula which is almost all drained into the IJV leading towards the heart (Fig. 20.7).

As time goes by if the ostium becomes wider, the haemodynamics then change substantially. Initially, as the forward flow of the artery proximal to the AVF maintains its pressure, an increasing amount of blood is lost via the fistula into the venous circulation. The forward arterial blood flow is then dramatically and progressively reduced (Fig. 20.8).

As the major leakage of the arterial blood occurs into the ostium, a certain proportion of the arterial blood having passed through the ostium, now travels cranially along the vein. This, for a vein, is a retrograde direction and results in stasis of the intracranial blood going towards the heart. This, in turn, leads to intracranial congestion and brain oedema. With the impedance to the cardiac flow of the blood along the IJV, the overall amount of cerebral venous blood going towards the heart is reduced (Fig. 20.9).

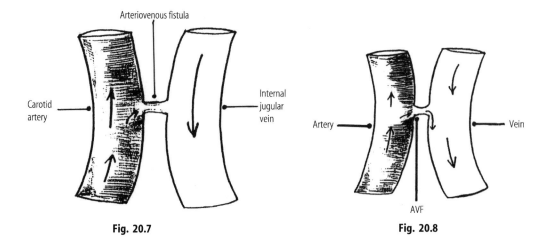

Fig. 20.7   **Fig. 20.8**

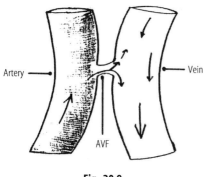

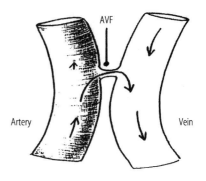

Fig. 20.9

Fig. 20.10

As the ostium enlarges even more, the greatest proportion of the arterial blood now leaks through the ostium making its way towards the heart (Fig. 20.10).

As the arterial blood turns towards the heart, by a Venturi effect, it pulls in, a greater portion of that blood of the artery which was intended for arterial forward flow (Fig. 20.11). So the carotid arterial flow is dramatically reduced distal to the level of the ostium. Over a period of time the proximal arterial flow is also correspondingly reduced because blood from a high resistance channel (artery) has leaked into a low resistance reservoir (vein). Poor venous resistance eventually contributes to a reduction of proximal arterial pressure as well (Fig. 20.12).

In such situations, since the greatest flow of the arterial blood is via the ostium towards the heart, the forward flow in the distal artery is almost negligible and the meagre amount is in fact pulled into the ostium by a Venturi effect (Fig. 20.13).

As a result of this abnormally directed blood flow, there is a tremendous turbulence produced. But this turbulence does not result in clot formation, because the blood is not allowed to stay for any great length of time. The fistula transmits a continuous arteriovenous machinery-type murmur and thrill, and may result in relative cerebral arterial deprivation on the side of the lesion. Because the fistula transmits a large quantity of arterial blood abnormally to the right side of the heart, the atrial filling pressure is substantially increased.

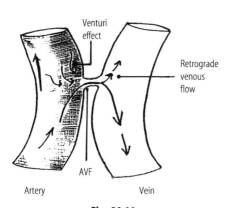

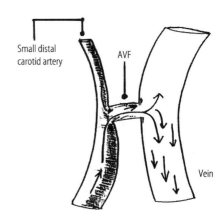

Fig. 20.11

Fig. 20.12

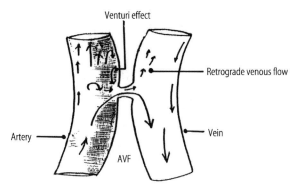

Fig. 20.13

If the fistula is mechanically occluded (by a finger), the suddenly reduced right atrial filling pressure results in the slowing down of the pulse rate and volume (Branham's sign). This sign can be easily demonstrated in the neck, but because of major haemodynamic fluctuations, this sign should not be repeatedly demonstrated.

An important general effect of such a caroticojugular fistula is a greater inload, resulting in congestive cardiac failure. Overall clinical disorders include congestive cardiac failure and cerebral congestive oedema of the ipsilateral side. In drastic situations, due to steal of arterial blood via the fistula, there may be a relative ipsilateral cerebral ischaemia produced as well.

With a proper history of trauma and correlating physical findings of a machinery-type murmur and an arteriovenous thrill, the diagnosis will be easy but it is essential to undertake proper dynamic and anatomical structural studies to evaluate the location and size of ostium, extent of collateral channels and the behaviour of the arteriovenous fistula.

A functional and dynamic study of an arteriovenous fistula can be undertaken by cineangiography or DSA. Cineangiography in two planes can give the appropriate information. If DSA is used then correct phases of the cineloop must be selected to reveal the ostium and the abnormal flow. The next step is to outline the distal artery and its diameter (a bypass graft may be necessary).

Another acceptable but slightly inferior investigation is cut film angiography, with pressure studies. Via an arterial catheter, pressures are measured in all of the four limbs of the AVF which gives a useful understanding of the haemodynamics, followed by conventional angiography in the arterial and in the venous phases (Fig. 20.14). Because of the presence of secondary cardiac failure, cardiac functional studies should also be undertaken, and this involves an assessment of the filling of the heart via echocardiogram, chest X-ray, electrocardiograms or if indicated, stress studies and cardiac catheterisation.

Of the general treatment of AVF of the neck, an essential requirement is concurrent correction of the cardiac failure by treatment with diuretics, cardiotonics and so on. If the patient's condition is not adequate, a preoperative cardiac therapy (to achieve the ideal status from the anaesthetic point of view), must be obtained. The general status of the patient is improved with correct nutrition and exercises.

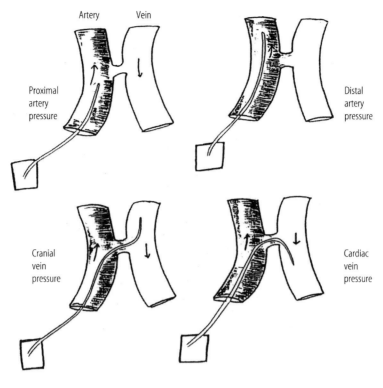

Fig. 20.14

Therapeutic embolisation using gelfoam or spring coils is a difficult procedure in the caroticojugular fistula because leakages from embolising material towards the heart or towards the cerebral hemisphere are dangerous. Also, any distortion of the carotid tree, at the site of implantation of the balloon, may produce platelet plug embolisations (TIAs). The main and the most relevant treatment is surgery. The area is explored in a way that the ostium is quickly located. Because of the fistulous communication, there is a preponderance of surface and superficial venous collateral channels present. This increases the local vascularity of the area imparting to it a greater heat and surgical risk during the exploration (Fig. 20.15).

A good method of dealing with these varicosities or abnormal venous involvements, is to ligate them as they are encountered in dissection, with ligaclips or fine suture materials methodically, before the AVF is dissected.

Once the peripheral vessels have been controlled then the carotid artery and the IJV above and below the fistula are identified, dissected clean, slung with vascular slings and prepared for clamping. Only after securing the four vessels relating to the fistula, is the fistula itself dissected free. In some situations it may be possible to isolate the fistula using the side-biting clamps, and partially occluding the IJV and the carotid artery (Fig. 20.16). But even in this situation, it is wise to secure the four vessels with vascular rubber slings first.

Then, having excised the fistula, lateral repair of both the carotid artery and the IJV is carried out using 5/0 Prolene for the artery, and 5/0 to 6/0 Prolene for the vein (Fig. 20.17a).

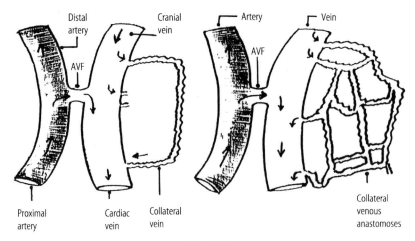

Fig. 20.15

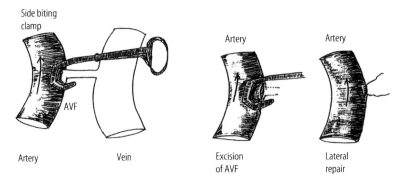

Fig. 20.16

Sandwiching a non-absorbable synthetic substance in between the artery and the vein (a vascular prosthetic patch), to prevent further AVF formation is controversial. As an alternative, the vascularised sternomastoid or sternohyoid can be rotated over the repair and interposed.

If lateral repair (of the artery and the vein) is not possible then vein patch or synthetic angioplasty (Fig. 20.17b) is performed to prevent stenosis. Alternatively bypass grafting of the affected vessels can be performed. Various kinds of non-absorbable, synthetic patch materials are available for this purpose, and a vascular patch (Vascutek) can be used to cover the vascular repair.

The reported results of vein angioplasty are superior and therefore vein patch graft is generally preferred. The results of the fistula excision and vascular repair are very good. As soon as the fistula is corrected, the heart rate and pulse volume reduce and the anaesthetist must be alert to this haemodynamic response. Pressor agents, colloid infusion, and so on, should be used immediately. Subsequently the heart adjusts to the reduced physiological input and the rhythm, rate and contractility become eventually normalised.

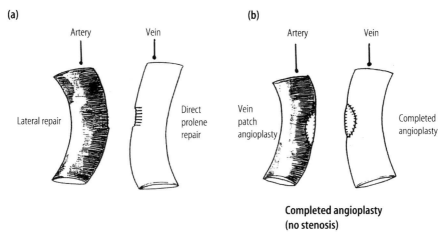

Fig. 20.17

20.5 Thrombosis of Carotid Sheath Vessels

Slow-onset delayed carotid arterial thrombosis usually occurs in elderly arteriopaths. Partial detachment or fracture of a plaque, is followed by progressive atherothrombosis, but the incidence of this disorder in the carotid artery is very much less than is seen in the region of the aortic bifurcation.

In the elderly, postangiographic occlusion of the ICA can occur if the ICA is already diseased significantly (90% or more). This is most probably due to activated clotting factors or due to reduced fibrinolytic capability, when the arterial intima is challenged by the hyperosmolar dye.[36–39]

Platelet-plug aggregation occurs at this nidus and the aggregate may form a secondary platelet plug. Localised thrombosis then follows and extends proximally and distally.

Traumatic arterial spasms and acute dissections can produce carotid thrombosis which usually occurs immediately after an injury (see sections 15.3 and 15.4). Rarely, the presence of an adjacent aneurysm or a loculated haematoma may gradually compress the artery over a long period of time, producing localised thrombosis. Whatever the mechanism, there is always a high probability of detached thrombi or new platelet aggregates embolising into the intracranial circulation (see sections 15.4 and 20.2).

IJV thrombosis may occur as a gradual process, by extension of a thrombus from a venous tributary. Cannulations for CVP measurements, parenteral nutrition, shunting (ventriculo-jugular shunts for hydrocephalus) or thoracic duct replantation procedures may result in gradual phlebitis and phlebothrombosis of the IJV.

The main danger from such a thrombus is development of a pulmonary embolism (PE). This should be actively prevented (see sections 15.4 and 19).

21 Thoracic Duct Injuries

On the left side the thoracic duct can be injured following a stab or a puncture injury to the root of the neck. Although largely fatal, the survivors of such penetrating injuries to the left subclavian triangle may sustain laceration or division of the thoracic duct in addition to more important and more dramatic soft tissue injuries. The structures at risk are the subclavian artery, internal jugualr vein (IJV), common carotid artery (CCA), roots of the brachial plexus, cervical dome of pleura and so on. Thoracic duct is much more commonly injured in the thorax (see Fig. 21.1).

Thoracic duct injuries

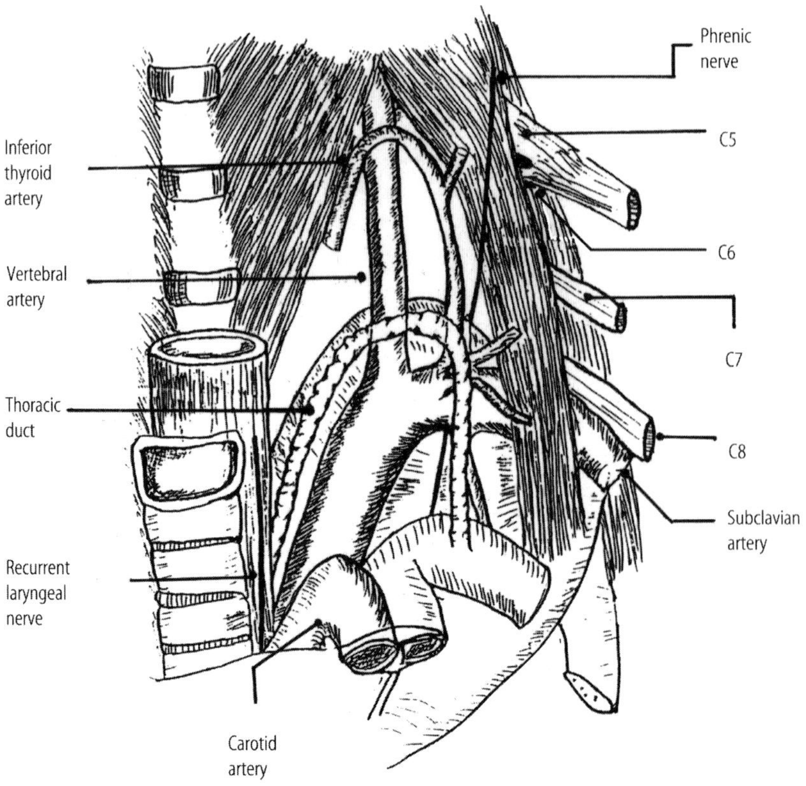

Fig. 21.1

21.1 Mechanisms of Thoracic Duct Injury

The thoracic duct can be injured iatrogenically during various types of surgical procedure intended for non-thoracic duct conditions, but an extrinsic non-surgical injury to the thoracic duct is almost always associated with neurovascular injuries. Thoracic duct injury can occur during an extensive gland exploration in the left supraclavicular fossa (as in block dissections). On yet rarer occasions misguided subclavian or internal jugular venous cannulations can result in an injury to the thoracic duct. It can also be damaged during a left-sided thoracic outlet decompression procedure especially during mobilisation of the second part of subclavian artery or during cervicodorsal sympathectomy.

21.2 Clinical Features of Thoracic Duct Injury and Management

Thoracic duct injury must be suspected when a chylous effusion leaks into the area following a regional injury. Without a significant injury, chylous effusion is very often associated with a malignancy. The output of the thoracic duct is chyle and this contains fat but this can easily be mistaken for pus. If the shiny fluid is examined on a glass slide, fat globules can be seen or the smear can be stained for fat, using Sudan III dye. The fluid can be examined biochemically as well, for its contents of cholesterol and triglycerides which will differentiate it from pus. A comparative assessment of the fluid against the patient's serum will show a greater level of cholesterol and triglyceride in the thoracic duct chyle. The electrophoresis of lipoprotein will reveal presence of chylomicrons present in chyle but not in serum. However, with a high index of suspicion and with careful visual inspection, the diagnosis of thoracic duct injury can be easily made and none of the elaborate tests are necessary except perhaps for confirmation.

Although rare now, thoracic duct discharge has been reported in sufferers of obstructive filariasis from endemically infested geographical areas. The transuded chyle from thoracic duct injuries should be differentiated from pseudochylous effusions which have a milky appearance and contain cholesterol and calcium phosphate crystals. Non-thoracic duct chyliform effusion contains fat and is derived from breakdown of cells of an encysted lesion. Differentiation between chylous and chyliform effusion is possible if lipophilic dyes are used. A suitable dye mixed with butter or milk is given by mouth. Twelve to 24 hours later, aspiration of the fluid is done and this will be coloured if the discharge is chylous. The dye commonly used for this purpose and to assist in the thoracic duct exploration is confectioners' green dye, known as DC-6.

The same technique should be used to identify a fistula of the thoracic duct during its exploration or postoperatively. A copious chylous effusion is secreted having a specific gravity of over 1.012. The fluid contains fat that can be separated with ether.

The majority of iatrogenic injuries tend to resolve with time and with conservative measures which include a low-fat diet. But if the area continues to ooze, it will produce metabolic disturbances and may result in a persisting discharging sinus that will become infected. In such conditions, appropriate investigations should be undertaken and the thoracic duct explored for repair, ligation or replantation.

Following an injury to the thoracic duct in the neck, effusion of 1.0–1.5 litres of chyle may take place in 24 hours, and therefore the patient will rapidly lose weight and become metabolically disturbed. If the thoracic duct is ligated then alternate collaterals may or may not satisfactorily drain the chyle into the venous system, but using microvascular techniques the injured thoracic duct can be replanted into an appropriate vein. A good recipient vein for the thoracic duct replantation is the external jugular vein.

21.3 Investigations of Thoracic Duct Injuries

Investigations should include a chest X-ray (thoracic inlet view) which may show a soft tissue expansion (chylous fluid) in the left subclavian triangle, or an apical pneumothorax representing an injury to the left pleural apex. Oral lipophilic dye (DC-6) can be given to stain the chylous effusion leaking from a fistula in the neck. Lymphangiography is not very useful in cervical thoracic duct injuries because it may fail to show leakages. Also, the lymphangiograms may take much longer to perform. Isotope imaging of the lymphatic duct can show an area of leakage but this investigation is more useful for mapping lymphatic channels and nodes in malignancy.

Enhanced computerised tomography (CT) scans can show a collection of large pools of chyle, but are not as useful as the isotope investigation. However, CT scanning is performed commonly to exclude a primary malignancy causing an obstructive chylous effusion. Such malignancies are more common in the chest and not in the neck.

The biochemistry of the transudate will show a high level of cholesterol and high specific gravity triglycerides. Cytology will show fat globules and chylomicrons from the transudate. Histology of the transudate and staining with Sudan III will show fat in the chyle. Metabolic investigation should be done to detect any secondary disorders relating to high lipid substance loss.

21.4 Treatment of Thoracic Duct Injuries

Conservative treatment includes reducing the pressure in the lymphatics by giving total parenteral nutrition for 2–3 weeks. An oral alternative, if the effusion is not substantial, is to give high carbohydrate, high protein fat-free diet in which periodic addition of medium-chain triglycerides can be made. The old-fashioned technique of pleurodesis to alter the pressure in the lymphatics has now been abandoned in favour of more direct treatment. The protein and the fat lost from the leakage should be replaced. Chylous effusion is often associated with local sepsis and a chest infection and these should be eradicated with use of appropriate antibiotics and drainage. The antibiotics of choice are those to whom the cultured bacteria are sensitive, but in practice these are likely to be a combination of third-generation cephalosporin and metronidazole or penicillin and gentamicin.

Usually, during an initial exploration, the commonest technique used is ligation of the divided end and some form of packing of the wound to abolish the dead space into which chyle accumulates. Even with simple one-stage ligation of the duct, collaterals usually form and make their way to the distal end of the duct or directly into an available vein. When this does not happen and if the leakage is substantial, progressive deterioration occurs with lipoprotein loss and recurrent infections. Repair and replantation should be done if microvascular surgical facilities and expertise are available. This should be done during the first exploration, since further surgery may encounter difficult adhesions and the results may not be as good as in primary repair.

Valved shunts can be incorporated in the replantation procedures, but these are of experimental nature and no major studies are available to suggest that these work better than a simple replantation procedure.

22 Sternomastoid and Scalene Muscular Injuries

Since the sternomastoid and scalene muscles overlie both the posterior as well as the anterior triangles, they are liable to injuries in a much larger surface area. The sternomastoid protects the carotid sheath and its injury is usually associated with additional more important injuries, such as to the carotid sheath, thyroid gland, roots and the trunks of brachial plexus, the IX, X and the XI cranial nerves.

Stabs and glass fragment injuries are common modes of penetrating injuries. Removal of *in situ* knife or glass results in renewed bleeding (see section 3). An obvious injury to the depth of the sternomastoid carries the same implications as penetration of peritoneum. Internal injuries cannot be excluded from a mere superficial inspection and formal exploration is mandatory.

The sternomastoid is a profusely vascularised muscle and tends to bleed extensively. The cut muscle fibres retract from the wound margins, in turn, retracting divided blood vessels. Individual cautery of bleeding points followed by mass haemostatic ligatures with chromic catgut (2/0) are necessary. After formal exploration for other more important injuries has been carried out with rectification, the muscle should be reattached using 3/4 interrupted deep chromic catgut. It is a functional and cosmetic muscle of the neck and serves as an important landmark for further surgery. Its loss may result in cosmetic asymmetry. Nerve supply is usually spared in most injuries.

The scalenus anterior muscle lies in a deeper compartment and is intimately related to the subclavian artery, its primary branches and to the roots of the brachial plexus. Phrenic nerve runs on its anteromedial aspect. The apex of the pleura is nearby.

Scalene injury is almost always associated with additional deep and important injuries to the neurovascular structures that should be systematically explored and dealt with. Following haemostasis of the scalenus anterior it should be haemostatically transected fully (by a cutting diathermy with due protection of the neurovascular structures). It is left divided to afford decompression against any ensuing deep plane compression that might occur due to fibrosis or adhesive organisation of haematoma.

Injuries to scalenus medius are associated with brachial plexus injuries and many of the blood vessels in the subclavian triangle may be injured. Direct haemostasis by ties and a formal regional exploration are necessary.

Injuries to the posterior nuchael muscles occur mainly due to blunt injuries. Occipital fractures and fractures of the cervical spine are being reported with increasing frequency with such injuries. Lacerations to the posterior longitudinal neck muscles are usually not life-threatening, except for those penetrating injuries which result in vertebral or spinal cord injuries. Following a fall, neurological examination and craniocervical X-rays (AP/Lat/Townes views) are necessary. The wound should be formally explored and haemostasis achieved by a combination of cautery and ties.

23 Injury to the Cervical Pleura

Accidental extrinsic penetrating neck injuries to the pleura are rare. Criminal injuries of the cervical pleura are relatively commoner. In the majority of cases a thoracic inlet penetrating injury forceful or deep enough to damage the pleura will inevitably result in major lacerations to the lung and other viscera of the neck or damage to the adjacent neurovascular structures. Many such injuries are accordingly fatal.

Iatrogenic pleural injuries may occur during block dissection of the neck, cervicodorsal sympathectomy or operations for thoracic outlet syndrome. Clavicular fractures are also associated with pleural injuries. The resultant pneumothorax is easily detectable and pleura should be properly repaired. The superficial area should be vacuum-drained. If the integrity of pleural repair is in any way doubtful, then a drain should be exteriorised for underwater drainage. In due course of time such injuries heal up fully, with mesothelial proliferation.

If severe bruising or lacerations of the apex of the corresponding lung is present this should be explored and repaired, if indicated, followed by underwater drainage.

24 Injury to Thyroid

Most thyroid injuries result from criminal stabs or from fragmented glass injuries in a car accident. Gunshot wounds are usually fatal. Attempted suicide and accidental falls resulting in thyroid cartilage injuries constitute a very small number. Iatrogenic injuries to the thyroid can occur during surgery and irradiation of the neck. Radiation damage to the thyroid can result in two major thyroid disorders:

● Hypothyroidism occurring after treatment of toxicosis with radioiodine.[47]

● Thyroid cancer. This is an independent side-effect of childhood irradiation. The incidence is within 20–100 cases per rad per million population. Similarly, parathyroid adenomas with abundant fibrosis can occur after therapeutic irradiations.[48]

The neck is a dangerously exposed area and the vital structures passing through it are at greater risk than at other locations (see Fig. 24.1).

Suicide attempts result in superficial platysmal injuries. Often anterior thyroid veins can be injured. Common facial and the external jugular veins are also thus exposed to slicing injuries. The ensuing bleeding is rarely life-threatening and can be easily controlled with external compression.

Puncture wounds (by spikes or knife points) and fragmented glass injuries can lacerate the anterior surface of thyroid lobe. A sharp injury to the lobe usually results in a continuous, but slow haemorrhage. Removal of the spike or glass may be followed by continuing

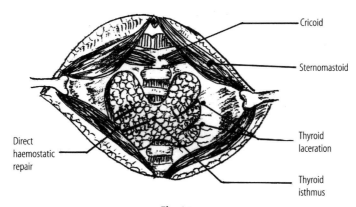

Fig. 24.1

arteriolar ooze that is prevented from discharging out by the sandwiching soft tissue. Haematoma thus builds up, producing laryngotracheal compression.

Associated injuries to the larynx or trachea may also be present, resulting in aspiration of blood, stridor and acute respiratory embarrassment.

The airway must be protected and as soon as the endotracheal or the nasotracheal tube is in position in the anaesthetised patient, a thorough exploration should be done, followed by direct haemostatic sutures of the thyroid lacerations. This usually suffices but often the thyroid vascular pedicles need to be formally ligated, as in standard partial thyroidectomy. It must be remembered that despite vascular pedicle ligatures, the lacerated thyroid may continue to bleed therefore it is logical to attempt direct haemostatic sutures of the lacerations (Fig. 24.1) first taking due care to prevent injuries to the recurrent laryngeal nerves.

Once haemostasis has been accomplished, trachea, larynx and adjacent structures are examined thoroughly. When this has been done adequately and no respiratory injury has been found on visual inspection, the anaesthetist should aspirate the throat and then deflate the cuff of the endotracheal tube. If still no air leaks are found then the tube is removed and detailed direct laryngoscopy is performed to ascertain any intrinsic damage, bleeding or perforation. If there is doubt about the integrity or if lacerations or perforations are seen on laryngoscopy then an immediate tracheostomy should be performed. A great majority of wounds in this region heal spontaneously under antibacterial cover if tracheostomy is performed and managed well. All thyroid injuries should be vacuum-drained using a reasonably sized tube. Ensuing pretracheal haematoma can thus be prevented from producing respiratory stridor. There should be no exception to this rule.

Concurrent tracheal or laryngeal injuries are relatively easy to detect, compared with oesophageal injuries.

Associated oesophageal injuries are rare but when these occur (blunt injuries, gunshot wounds, etc.), they produce a great misery. A good policy therefore is that if concurrent with thyroid injury a laryngotracheal injury is present then oesophageal puncture should also be suspected. An immediate gastrografin swallow screening or endoscopy should be done. If a tear is found, it should be repaired at once.

An endoscopy may show extensive bruising of the oesophagus and this usually indicates partial thickness oesophageal injury. With detection of minor oesophageal injuries a double lumen nasogastric tube should be implanted. Continuous low pressure suction will keep the stomach empty and the side channels of the tube will aspirate saliva and so on. If infection is prevented then spontaneous healing usually follows.

Concurrent with thyroid injuries if obvious mediastinitis is present then proper underwater drainage should be established, in addition to repairing the oesophageal tear. However, on rare occasions, cases have been reported when oesophageal injury occurs only in the neck and the thoracic oesophagus is spared. Obviously in such a situation if access is possible to intact oesophagus above and below the tear then a simple repair in the neck should be done followed by local drainage and antibiotic cover. Use of stents (to prevent stenosis) is not very popular in cervical oesophageal injuries where primary repair can be adequately done without producing a stricture.

If deep multiple thyroid injuries are present (shotgun pellets, glass fragments or multiple stabs) then additional injuries must be suspected to the vascular structures, Recurrent laryngeal nerves, trachea, larynx, oesophagus, pharynx, etc.). In addition to exploration and haemostasis of the thyroid, a protective temporary tracheostomy should be seriously considered. The area should be drained and appropriate prophylactic antibiotics must be given.

25 Injury to Cranial Nerves in the Neck

Isolated injuries to the cranial nerves following external cervical trauma are rare. Usually, an injury severe enough to cause cranial nerve damage is fatal. Among the survivors such a cranial nerve injury is usually found with more important concomitant injuries such as to the vessels, trachea, oesophagus or spinal cord. Isolated cranial nerve injuries in the neck are much more commonly produced by iatrogenic trauma.

The hypoglossal nerve is occasionally damaged while dissecting the internal carotid artery during elective carotid endarterectomy. The vagus nerve can be damaged during dissections for excision of a carotid body tumour, carotid sheath injuries or hurried attempts at haemostasis during a block dissection. The spinal accessory nerve may get injured with stabs to the neck penetrating the sternomastoid muscle. Its loss does not result in a major functional deficit.

Iatrogenic injuries to the cervical branch of the facial nerve can occur during a difficult dissection of the submandibular gland. Similarly, dissections around the parotid gland may result in a damage to the facial nerve.

Maxillofacial fractures associated with neck injuries may disrupt the main VII nerve. If evidence exists of injuries to lower cranial nerves, then it is more likely for the neck injury to be associated with the fracture of the base of the skull. A full and formal neurological examination is essential, supported by good X-rays and a computed tomography (CT) or a magnetic resonance imaging (MRI) scan.

Chiropractic injuries (therapeutic manipulations of the cervical spine) may produce neuropraxia of the X nerve or spinal shock, in addition to bony vertebral injuries and vertebral artery thrombosis.

An essential part of the management includes protection of neck from further injuries. The neck, after a closed injury should be adequately splinted or be encased in a soft cervical collar for safe transportation before X-rays are taken to determine fractures of the craniocervical region. A CT scan also helps in the location of traumatic syringomyelia and haemorrhage.

26 Injuries to the Cervical Spine and the Spinal Cord

Blunt injuries to the neck can cause vertebral disruptions resulting in damage to spinal cord. Such cord damage can range from minor bruising to transection. Therefore, symptomatology may range between neurogenic shock and paralysis. Ordinarily, the degree of violence has to be considerable, to injure the spinal cord but when the neck is unguarded (under anaesthesia, car accidents, whiplash injuries, etc.), seemingly trivial forces can disrupt the spinal cord!

Most such injuries occur in young people (males more often than females; average age of 25 years) and involve aggressive activities such as sport injuries, car accidents, falls and assaults.

A rough universal annual estimate of 10,000 new cases of acute spinal cord injuries is reasonable. Isolated cervical spine injuries are however uncommon. They usually occur nowadays, with road traffic accidents (RTAs), and head and limbs are often concomitantly involved. Although isolated spinal injuries are rare, their presence warrants a very aggressive early management, if major disability or loss of life is to be avoided.

Any cervical vertebra can be injured with violence. Interesting eponyms have been historically allocated to peculiar vertebral injuries.

"Jefferson's fracture" is a bilateral bursting fracture of anterior and posterior arches of C_1 against the occipital condyles. An axial loading from the top of the skull can produce such an injury. The "hangman's fracture", encountered in judicial hanging and hyperextension injury, relates to fracture of the pedicles of C_2 with subluxation of C_2 on C_3, resulting in spinal shock, transection or avulsion of the cord. Traditionally, a 1–2 metre drop with a noose around the neck results in an initial spinal shock and death from strangulation and asphyxia. A drop of more than 2 metres, almost always snaps vertebrae (most commonly the C_2) resulting in cord avulsion. "Clay shoveller's fracture" is a form of fatigue fracture of spinous processes of lower cervical vertebrae (below C_3) caused by direct trauma or muscular exertion in labourers.[45]

In rheumatoid arthritis the apposed facets are fused due to spondylosis, ageing or demineralisation, and repeated stress during shovelling and so on, snaps up the facets or the pedicles producing a small fracture difficult to identify with conventional views of X-rays of the cervical spine. MRI scans are more reliable for diagnosis.

Odontoid fracture can occur from falls, blows to the skull, road accidents and sport injuries. These are divided into three types:

●   Type 1 is a fracture throught the tip of the odontoid process.

●   Type 2 is a fracture through the body of the process.

●   Type 3 is a fracture through the base and the body of C_2.

Shallow water diving injuries can result in severe hyperflexion and dislocation of cervical spine at any level.

RTA deceleration can produce a whiplashing injury of the neck at various levels. As the car suddenly comes to a stop in an accident, the body continues to move forward. This deceleration is prevented by the activated inertia seat-belt that locks the shoulder strap and the lap belt. However, the restraining effects of the safety belt are confined to the trunk and to the pelvis. The neck continues to decelerate forwards in its upper part. Acute cervical flexion with stretching, is thus transiently produced (Fig. 26.1a). This is followed suddenly by the recoiling of the neck backwards by the protective reflexes, like the lash of a whip! (Fig. 26.1b).

The force of the whiplash manoeuvre can transmit severe pressure to the atlantoaxial ligaments (the reflex recoil sends the head backward on a fixed thorax). The result may be a fracture of the odontoid process of the C_2 with dislocation, resulting in crushing of the spinal cord. A whiplash is a biphasic injury, when opposing forces work against each other. This is not merely a hyperextension injury of the cervical spine.[49] The introduction of a fixed or adjustable headrest has prevented many injuries. Reflex hyperextension is prevented by the headrest during the whiplashing (Fig. 26.2).

Modern cars are fitted with air-bag systems for driver and front-seat passenger and these have dramatically reduced the incidence of whiplash injuries. Soon, "smart" air-bags which adjust to body size for children and to force of impact, are expected to be installed routinely.

(a)   (b)

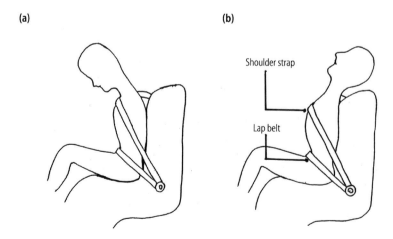

Fig. 26.1

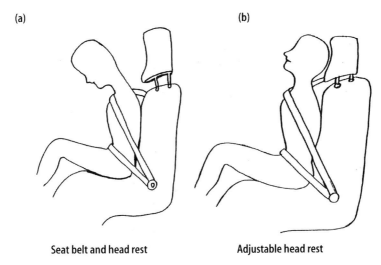

(a)   (b)

Seat belt and head rest   Adjustable head rest

Fig. 26.2

Diving injuries or accidental falls on the head can result in the impaction of cervical spinal cord on itself. The lower cord can be directly crushed or the fractured pieces of bones can impale the cord from above, resulting in transection.

Penetrating injuries of the cervical spinal cord are almost always caused by a high velocity missile (rifle bullet from 10–20 metres or a pistol bullet from a closer range). The bullet can track through to the pedicles or to the disc space. The secondary missile effect of the fragmented bone and dense tissue (disc, ligaments) can easily cause an injury to the cord, possibly some distance away from the track itself. This is the main mechanism of the bullet injuries to the cord. The blast and the shockwave effects do not contribute much by way of cord damage. Cavitation effect also does not seem to cause much damage to the cord itself (see sections 4.2.3 and 4.2.4). Occasionally a bullet entering the neck from an anterolateral direction can ricochet against the transverse processes or pedicles and can come to rest against the spinal cord in the spinal canal, causing local compression to the cord at that level. An urgent decompression must be done with removal of bullet to salvage the cord.

The force of shotgun pellets is much too small to penetrate to the depth of the spinal cord but close range injuries (less than 5 metres) can cause destruction of the cord by a few pellets. This is almost always fatal (see section 4.3).

Blast and explosion injuries tend to produce relatively greater damage to the middle and to the internal ear, eustachian tubes and to hollow viscera, but spinal cord injury has also been reported. Much more numerous are shrapnel neck injuries, encountered with bomb explosions, resulting in penetrating injuries to the spinal cord.

When initial cervical spine injury occurs, some of the damage is probably reversible. It is this aspect which is often made worse with mishandling and with bad transport. Transportation should be conducted in an organised way to minimise such injuries and to preserve intact tissue. At its simplest a soft collar can protect the injured neck during short transport, but where it is deemed that external immobilisation might be the definitive treatment then the following collars and supports can be used from the start:

- Philadelphia collar. This is a strengthened semi-rigid foam brace that prevents flexion and extension, but allows some rotation.

- Miami-J collar. This is a similar synthetic device that provides greater stiffness and additional padding.

- Thermoplastic Minerva body jacket. The TMBJ is a brace that can immobilise an unstable fracture. It allows less flexion and extension at each intervertebral level and yet provide some comfort.

- Halo vest. This allows significantly less overall rotation than the TMBJ.

- Sterno-occipito-mandibular immobilizer. The SOMI can be used as an external supporting device for stable fractures. The four poster or the Yale brace are other alternatives.

Patients can be lifted with such support on to a stretcher and then on to a Stryker turning frame. At its simplest, Glissons slings, wrapped around the patient's chin can be applied and traction, should commence immediately during transportation, to stabilise the injured spine.[50] In general, 2.25 kg (5 lb) of weight per level of injury, allowing 3 kg (7 lb) for the weight of the skull should be used. With this rule of thumb a C_5–C_6 injury should be treated with 13.5–16 kg (30–35 lb) of traction. However, this may not suffice with partial cord transection or displaced and unstable vertebral injuries. In such situations, under local anaesthesia, a skull calliper can be applied without drilling (Gardner Wells system does not require drilling of the outer table) or with a central drill using the Blackburn or the Crutchfield tongs.[28]

The dislocated spine should be reduced as soon as possible, preferably within the first few hours of trauma.[51,52] This can be done under a general anaesthesia or even light sedation using traction weights gradually increasing to 18–20 kg (40–50 lb). Once reduction has been achieved and confirmed radiologically, the weight can be reduced by 2.25–3 kg (5–7 lb).[53] Over-distraction must be prevented. Spinal cord oedema which adds insult to injury must be prevented and treated:

- Methylprednisolone crosses the cell membrane rapidly and improves the outcome if used within 8 hours of injury (bolus of 30 mg/kg followed by an infusion of 5.4 mg/kg over 23 hours. Antacids and H_2-receptor antagonists also have a place.

- Tirilizad mesylate through its antioxidant activity without the glucocorticoid action can improve the injury.

- GM-1 ganglioside, an acidic glycolipid with neuroprotective and restorative potential is under study (100 mg of GM-1 within 72 hours followed by a lower maintenance dose for 3–4 weeks).

The use of dimethyl sulfoxide (DMSO) is gaining popularity in the recovery from experimental trauma to the central nervous system (CNS) in animals, but no clinical trials in live human subjects has yet been reported. DMSO reduces inflammatory response and promotes osmotic diuresis.[54]

DMSO also improves microcirculation[55] by:

● inhibiting platelet aggregation through an increase in the cAMP and a corresponding decrease in the phosphodiesterase

● direct vasodilatation from increased PGE_1 (vasodilator) and inhibition of PGF_2 and PGE_2 (vasoconstrictors).

Peripheral nerve transfer has already been used to bridge the area of cord injury. These grafts have a specific advantage in that the Schwann cells can form pathways for axonal growth and do not encourage glial scars. This has successfully been undertaken in dogs[56] and rats. [57] Successful transplantation of cortical tissue in the area of cord hemitransection has already been reported in mammals.[58]

27 Brachial Plexus Injuries

The most common mechanism of injury is an unguarded fall of a motorcyclist on an outstretched hand. The fall produces a shearing injury by traction, to the brachial plexus (BP). Such a traumatic mechanism produces all grades of injuries ranging from neuropraxia to axonotmesis and rupture by avulsion of the roots from the spinal cord (see Fig. 27.1). The lesions can be grouped as upper, lower and total in respect of root values:

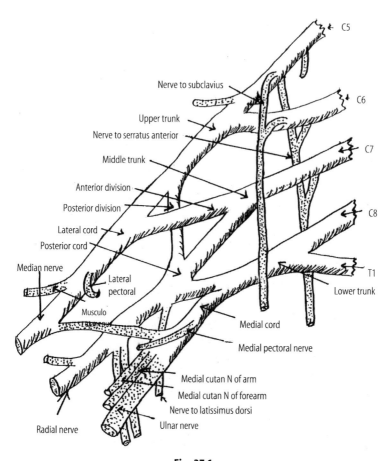

Fig. 27.1

- upper BP lesions involve $C_{(4),5,6,7}$ roots.

- lower BP lesions involve C_8 and T_1 roots

- total BP lesion involves the roots of the entire plexus ($C_{(4),5}$–T_1).

Other less common injuries to the brachial plexus arise from penetrating trauma caused by gunshot wounds. The bullet can severe BP roots, trunks or their divisions, in the supra-clavicular region. Even if no actual contact is made between the bullet and the nerves, the vibratory, thermal or shockwave effects of the passing missile can damage these nerves. Penetrating and sharp injuries are more easily treatable than indirect ones, because the ends of the nerve may be close by, and may not be associated with a large gap.

Knife injuries to the side of the neck (supraclavicular fossa) can severe roots and trunks of the BP. Such injuries are relatively more easy to repair than traction injuries where the extent of the nerve loss may be much more severe. Glass injuries can cause similar damage to the BP but their removal results in a further or "second" injury (see section 3.2). Removal of *in situ* glass should therefore be only undertaken during a planned formal exploration. Glass leads to the site of the damage and the exploration has a better chance of locating and repairing the damaged nerves primarily.

Blunt injuries to the BP can occur through clavicular fracture. Considering that clavicular fractures are quite common, resultant BP injuries are surprisingly rare. When these occur in association with a rifle injury then secondary missile effect can cause serious widespread injury. Deceleration road traffic accident injuries and compression injuries (steering wheel injuries to the driver) can cause serious BP injuries by penetration of in-driven bony fragments.

Open injuries to BP (penetration by knife, bullet, glass, secondary missile effect of bone, debris and tissue fragment) are almost always associated with additional internal injuries such as to the corresponding lung, pleura, blood vessels, cranial nerves or spinal cord.[43,46] Therefore, a full assessment for an overall management is imperative. Only the motorcyclist's brachial plexus syndrome (loss of functions of the nerves of the BP) is known to occur in isolation. In this condition there may be total avulsion of various parts of the BP without an obvious external injury. The helmet protects the head, but the dangerously exposed arms are easily injured in the ensuing twisting fall, encountered with skidding, slipping or falling from the motorcycle.

Unless life appears to be in jeopardy (when resuscitation should take first priority), a thorough neurological assessment must be made. The injuries and the overall condition of the patient should be assessed, investigated and documented. Lung and vascular lesions take priority.

Once loss of neurological function is detected, spinal cord injury should be suspected until disproved, and undue neck movement avoided. Once spinal cord lesion has been excluded (and this may take some time since BP neurological manifestations may mimic spinal cord lesion and vice versa), then the BP should be treated. If skin loss has occurred or contamination is obviously present then wound closure by primary skin suture is best avoided. The wound is cleaned, debrided and dressed, and in due course of time skin graft or delayed primary sutures of the skin can be performed. If the exterior is infected or if abundant foreign bodies have been introduced, then any BP repairs will be subjected to infective processes and will most certainly fail. The therapeutic approach should then be more conservative in the first instance. In stab injuries to the BP, as soon as primary skin sutures have healed (about 2 weeks later), BP repair can be undertaken.

In rare presentations when the wound is surgically clean and tidy, if the general condition of the patient is good then primary repair of the BP should be undertaken, if facilities and expertise are available. If these clinical parameters are not up to scratch then in the interest of the patient, the skin should be closed and the patient transferred to an appropriate unit for further treatment. If a vascular injury is present then urgent exploration for haemostasis and vascular salvage must be undertaken. This provides as good a time as any, for primary BP repair as well,[43] if the injury is relatively "clean". It should be remembered that the first repair is the best repair, and a primary repair soon after the injury provides good landmarks and offers to the patient the best chance of function-restoration.

If primary repair is to be undertaken then this should be preceded by formal investigations and preparations. This, therefore, implies that the patient has actually presented to a specialist unit directly. There is considerable wisdom, in the author's opinion, in a majority of cases, to postpone the BP exploration for 2–3 weeks. In this period of time, the condition of the patient becomes stabilised and good neurological work-up can be done to diagnose and to locate the level of the injury. Such work-up includes neurophysiological assessment and may include cervicocranial computerised tomography (CT) scans or nuclear magnetic resonance (NMR) (magnetic resonance imaging, MRI) scans. Nerve conduction velocities (NCV) and somatosensory evoked potentials (SEPs) should be done accurately and bilaterally for assessment and to form a baseline. Associated treatment (plating of fractures) can also be planned during this waiting or observation period. If evidence points to the possibility of a spinal cord lesion or a very high root lesion then CT cervical myelography should be carried out. If a myelocele is seen adjacent to a particular nerve root then the avulsion of the BP root will be considered as complete and therefore no specific repair can or should be undertaken except for selective neurotisations. In closed injuries to the BP (brachial plexus syndrome), since the skin is intact and no exogenous infection is introduced, a primary exploration and repair give the best results.

One of the main problems with closed BP nerve injuries (especially traction injuries) is persistent functional nerve deficit in presence of an anatomically intact nerve. In such situations, the nerve seemingly looks intact but has internal axonal disruption, fibrosis and resultant conduction block. This is called a "lesion-in-continuity". The essential part of treatment is to intraoperatively stimulate the uninjured proximal part of the involved nerve and to record a nerve action potential (NAP) across the site of injury. If NAPs are obtained (positive) across the damaged segment, then enough axonal connection persists to allow eventual recovery and therefore this nerve should either be just left alone or be just neurolysed from intra- and extra-epineurial fibrosis. If on the other hand, proximal stimulation fails to produce an NAP across the area of damage, then no matter how clinically intact the damaged segment looks, it must be resected and the defect bridged by a graft such as from the sural nerve.[59,60]

27.1 Functional Grouping of BP lesions

Functionally, BP lesions are grouped together as follows.

27.1.1 Proximal Palsy

Here the upper trunk alone is damaged. The lesion of C_{5-6} produces a loss of shoulder joint movements and elbow flexion. Hand movements are preserved.

27.1.2 Proximal Palsy with Radial Nerve Involvement

The lesion mimics the proximal palsy of the upper trunk but is associated with a wrist drop (C_{5-7}).

27.1.3 Distal Palsy

The C_8-T_1 lesion produces hand weakness (not total paralysis). Shoulder and elbow functions may or may not be affected.

27.1.4. Total Palsy

The root lesions C_5-T_1 produce total sensory and motor deficit of the upper limb.

27.1.5 Mixed Lesion

In this type of injury, patchy lesions not conforming to an identifiable pattern, are present. This may be present in association with the BP lesion due to an associated high cervical sympathetic chain disruption.

The best site for external stimulation of the nerve trunks of the BP is from the Erb's point. This is located just above the clavicle lateral to the lateral edge of the clavicular head of sternomastoid corresponding to the level of the sixth cervical vertebra. (The site of origin of the suprascapular nerve from the upper trunk is also known as the Erb's point.)

Systematic recordings are taken of evoked muscle action potentials following stimulation of specific nerves for proximal muscles (musculocutaneous nerve for biceps, suprascapular nerve for supraspinatus and infraspinatus, circumflex nerve for deltoid, radial nerve for triceps). The recording needle electrodes (G1) are placed in the belly of each muscle (sometimes at different levels along a vertical line in the middle of a single muscle).

(a)   (b)

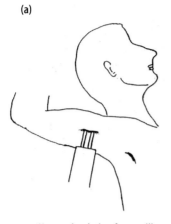

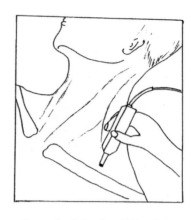

Nerve stimulation from axilla   Nerve stimulation from Erb's point

Fig. 27.2

Distances from Erb's point to G1 are measured with a calliper (Fig. 27.2). Normal mean latencies are then worked out and documented.

27.2 Normal Mean Latencies

Normal mean latencies are listed in Table 27.1.

Table 27.1 Normal mean latencies

Muscle	Distance from Erb's point (cm)	Latency (ms)
Biceps	20.0	4.6
Deltoid	15.5	4.3
Triceps	21.5	4.5
Supraspinatus	8.5	2.6
Infraspinatus	14.0	3.4

27.3 Repair Options

The options of repair are as follows.

27.3.1 Neurolysis

Neurolysis of adherent and entrapped nerves, usually the trunks can be done in two ways:

- *External neurolysis* can expedite subsequent recovery of function.[61,62] In this procedure, the adherent nerve sheath is carefully separated from the surrounding tissue by sharp dissection so as to remove all tension, stretch, kinking and compression.

- *Internal neurolysis* can be performed by saline injections through a microneedle under magnification (using an operating microscope) to loosen the adherent fascicles from the sheath and perineurium. There is now some controversy about its role.[63] The author has found this to be quite useful, but since internal neurolysis is almost always performed in conjunction with external neurolysis, it is difficult to validate its specific role.

Whichever form of neurolysis is done, the procedure should be guided by an intraoperative nerve action potential (NAP) recording. If, in a lesion-in-continuity, NAPs are positive then a simple neurolysis rather than complicated grafting, should produce about 90% function–restoration.[64]

27.3.2 Primary Repair

This involves direct suture of divided nerve ends. This can only be done in almost surgical wounds (clean stabs). Such a neurorrhaphy must only be undertaken if there is no tension present in the anastomosis. Results are better than grafting.

27.3.3 Grafting

Grafting involves obtaining a length of sural nerve, superficial radial nerve, or in exceptional circumstances, an adjacent nerve. This can be anastomosed using very fine sutures or by fibrin glue between the two divided ends.

27.3.4 Nerve Transfer

This can be done by sacrificing one nerve for another at the local site (neurotisation). The spinal accessory nerve is very useful for neurotisation. Since the injury to the nerve can occur at more than one level, there may be avulsion injuries sustained to the brachial plexus roots and trunks and there might be additional nerve injuries present distally, such as to the circumflex nerve at the surgical neck of the humerus, or to the radial nerve in the spiral groove.

A comprehensive assessment must be made as thoroughly as possible.

27.4 Management Protocol

The author's protocol for the management of BP injuries includes the following.

1 A quick clinical assessment of the overall condition with particular emphasis to the spinal cord, respiration and the local blood vessels. Spinal cord injury demands use of a cervical collar or supportive traction immediately, followed by gently performed X-rays, CT scans or NMR (MRI) scans. Tracheal or laryngeal injuries require a tracheostomy followed by local repair. Vascular injuries require immediate safe haemostasis and volume restoration.

2 After an initial and immediate assessment of vital signs and the features mentioned above, a thorough assessment of the overlying skin, introduced infection, state of the pleura and lung, stabilisation of an associated arm or clavicular fracture, Chest X-ray in expiration (to outline pneumothorax) and X-rays of a suspected limb fracture must be performed rapidly.

3 Where a positive neurological finding is present or when a neurospinal injury is suspected, a detailed neurological mapping of the lesion with bilateral comparison and documentation must be performed. Nerve conduction velocities (NCV) from Erb's point stimulation and somatosensory evoked potentials (SEP) where root avulsion is suspected, should be performed. In selected cases a CT cervical myelography or a MRI scan to exclude a high root lesion (by the presence of a myelocele) should be performed.

4 If no contraindication exists for an operation (such as contaminated wound, major skin loss, laryngotracheal injuries, associated head or chest injuries, suspected seat-belt abdominal injuries), then preoperative preparations can begin. If a contraindication to surgery exists then the operation on the BP is postponed. When this is undertaken electively, then in addition to an overall assessment again (as described above), up to 4 units of blood are arranged. An informed consent is taken at which time the details of the operation and the likely predicted outcome is clearly explained to the patient. Total body disinfection with chlorhexidine is undertaken with depilation of the corresponding axilla and both lower legs. With anaesthetic induction, a fast-acting intravenous cephalosporin (duly skin tested), is administered.

5 At the time of exploration, an NAP recording facility is essential. The exposure must be very elaborate and nerves above and below must be clearly identified at the time of surgery. Documentation with measurements and photographs should also be made.

6 When an operable BP syndrome is strongly suspected, the surgeon must assume that at least some of the divided nerves will require nerve grafting and therefore it is best to start off with harvesting of the donor sural nerves. The patient is therefore intubated, paralysed and positioned in a prone position. Under a tourniquet control, the sural nerve from one or both sides is harvested and soaked in normal saline awaiting grafting. The wound is closed, dressed and the patient turned over to supine position. Drapes, instruments, gloves and swabs are changed. The author prefers to keep the patient's affected arm by the side at 20°. This allows a certain degree of lowering of the clavicle and of increasing access in the supraclavicular fossa. A semi-sitting posture is also very useful, but this imposes certain anaesthetic difficulties and accordingly a supine position is preferred by most surgeons and anaesthetists. The head is turned to the opposite side.

For penetrating injuries, a transverse supraclavicular approach offers the best and the quickest access to the roots and trunks of the BP.

For closed injuries, a much more elaborate exposure may become necessary and therefore a supraclavicular incision going across the clavicle, via the deltopectoral groove, to the axilla, offers a very good access. The clavicle can be divided and with lateral retraction of the lateral half of the clavicle, the plexus can be followed into the axilla. Anatomical orientation should be aided by liberal use of the nerve stimulator. If clavicular osteotomy is deemed necessary then plate holes are drilled first, before performing clavicular osteotomy. subclavian vein must be preserved during this procedure.

When the transected nerve is found, the gap is measured, a photograph is taken and its ends are freshened with a knife. The cut ends are inspected with an operating microscope or a powerful loupe. The landmarks of tiny blood vessels or bundles of fibres help to orientate the nerve. A mismatch results in severe loss of function. With proper matching and orientation, the intrafascicular stitch anchors the nerve at one or two points. Four to eight interrupted sutures are enough to reapproximate the nerve sheath without undue tension. This is a primary repair of the native nerve achieved through some mobilisation of the nerve segment. However, neurorrhaphy must only be performed if no tension is present at the site of anastomosis (Fig. 27.3). When there is doubt, a nerve graft must be interposed[65-68] and anchored by sutures in a similar manner or by using tissue glue (fibrin glue).

In the majority of cases, such an easy primary neurorrhaphy is not possible. The nerve ends either develop an ungraftable neuroma requiring local excision or the ends undergo reaction of degeneration (RD). In such situations, the wasted portion of the nerve must be transected, the ends freshened and grafted to sural nerve strands. (If the nerve ends cannot be brought together for anastomosis, despite bracing and lifting of the shoulder, then sural nerve interposition grafting should be performed.)

If the length of the sural nerve is adequate for the desired graft then full diameter grafts are made using the operating microscope. If the available length of the sural nerve is short, then strands of sural nerve are cut and used as grafts.

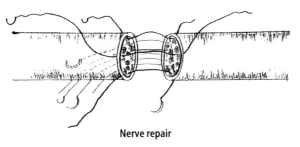

Nerve repair

Fig. 27.3

The preferred recipient nerves for grafting are the median, ulnar and radial nerves in this order, but the musculocutaneous nerve should also be grafted if possible for salvage of elbow functions.

The anastomotic sites should be protected from adhesive entrapment and therefore grafts should be routed away from inflamed sites, haematoma cavities and so on. Sleeves of silastic tubing or vascular tubular externally reinforced graft (Goretex or Vascutek) can be used to isolate the vulnerable areas, but most surgeons do not like using synthetic material near the nerve anastomoses for fear of infection and rejection. Since the increased prevalence of AIDS, use of biological glue has become much less popular.

When all of the severed nerves are anastomosed the wound is irrigated with saline. Some surgeons like dusting with antibiotic spray (Neomycin, streptomycin, polymyxin). The elbow is splinted in a functional position. Wrist drop is corrected by an extension of the forearm splint or by application of a detachable wrist splint supported by velcrose.

A drain is avoided for fear of introducing infection, therefore haemostasis should be very good without a tourniquet. After removal of skin sutures, passive mobilisation begins, to prevent contractures.

Three months later, repeat nerve conduction velocities and somatosensory evoked potentials (NCVs, SEPs) help to show some degree of reinnervation. A common finding at this stage is the absence of denervation-fibrillations. An active course of physiotherapy followed by occupational therapy should be started and continued indefinitely. The final recovery may take several months and the patients must be adequately supervised in the interim.

The final outcome of the BP repair may be less than perfect but if repair is not attempted, there will be no useful spontaneous improvement forthcoming. If the patient is young and if the injury is fresh, the results are likely to be much better.

If during exploration, the outlook does not appear to be very encouraging, then neurotisation, using the spinal accessory nerve or even transposition of muscles should be considered to allow wrist extension and elbow flexion. Innervated latissimus dorsi rotation and osteosynthesis or fusion of the wrist joint in a neutral position can benefit the patient in selected cases.

The published results of BP repairs are grossly variable but functional salvage is only achieved if an aggressive attitude is adopted by the surgeon. The younger the patient the better the results. Since the first repair offers the best results, where a primary repair is indicated, this should be undertaken soon by an experienced surgeon to achieve the best salvage.

28 General Features of Injuries to the Larynx, Trachea and Oesophagus

The two major threats to life following a penetrating injury to the neck are airway obstruction and bleeding. Early exploration and appropriate repair is essential.[69] The main cause of death in such injuries is obstruction to the upper airway. Attention should be given to the establishment of an airway even before the arrest of haemorrhage, except in rare specific situations. If respiratory salvage is delayed to the point of central cyanosis, which is a sign of impending death (not a sign of respiratory obstruction), this could be too late. Noisy breathing is obstructed breathing, however, when the obstruction is total, there would be no noise present![70] No patient with questionable airway obstruction should be given an analgesic with a potential for respiratory depression.[70]

Visceral injuries of the neck are more common than expected. Neurovascular injuries show their manifestations dramatically and may divert the attention of the clinician away from the visceral injuries. An obvious laryngeal penetrating injury produced by a stab or by a bullet is life threatening and easy to detect, but a minor laryngeal or oesophageal injury may not be easy to detect on initial presentation. Laryngeal injuries may be concealed and may require an indirect (endoscopic) or direct (thyrotomy) assessment. Panendoscopy of hypopharynx, laryngotracheal region and oesophagoscopy must be undertaken even if just a single viscus appears to be injured.

Maintenance of respiratory functions and haemostasis are key factors in the functional salvage of the patient.

When multiple injuries of the neck are present such as in road traffic accidents (RTAs) or shotgun trauma, then nothing short of cricothyroidostomy or tracheostomy should be considered in the first instance as an initial part of resuscitation.

Respiratory access and salvage may range from airway protection to tracheostomy. "In-between" procedures include orotracheal or nasotracheal intubation and cricothyroidostomy (by needle puncture or division of cricothyroid membrane) and minitracheostomy.

Puncture cricothyroidostomy can be quickly performed using two large bore cannulae. Through one, oxygen can be administered and through the other the expirate can be vented. "Mini trach", a modified form of short-cut tracheostomy is a much better technique than cricothyroidostomy.

In RTAs, maxillofacial injuries may complicate neck injuries and respiratory salvage assumes a paramount position in the overall management.

Since cricothyroidostomy and tracheostomy are the mainstay of management and must precede surgical repair of most of the laryngeal and tracheal injuries, these procedures are described here first.

29 Cricothyroidostomy

This is a reliable and fast method of providing an airway through the trachea. Clinically, the neck is palpated anteriorly and cricothyroid membrane is located (the space between the cricoid cartilage and the thyroid lower border is the cricothyroid space and in this thyroid–cricoid interspace the cricothyroid membrane lies subcutaneously). To palpate it properly, the thyroid cartilage is first stabilised with two fingers and then an index finger is inserted into the thyroid–cricoid interspace (Fig. 29.1). Once this has been established then the procedure of cricothyroidostomy can begin (Fig. 29.2).

With the patient lying supine a small area anteriorly, in the region of proposed cricothyroidostomy, is prepared antiseptically and is injected with local anaesthetic.

It is better to mark the site of the incision with indelible ink so that the obliteration of the landmark with the infiltration of the local anaesthetic can be avoided; 1:100,000 adrenaline and 1% lignocaine 5 ml is injected into various planes of cricothyroid space. When the area has been antiseptically prepared with povidone iodine, chlorhexidine and so on, then towels and drapes (opsite adhesive drape) can be applied to isolate the area. In desperate situations

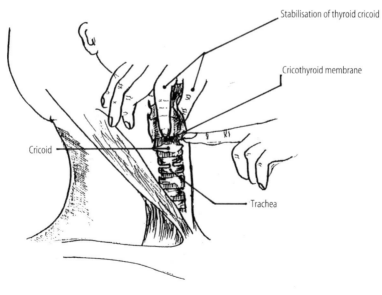

Fig. 29.1

115

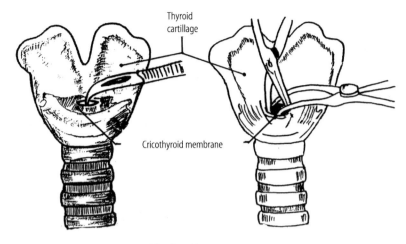

Cricothyroidostomy

Fig. 29.2

no antisepsis or formal preparation is required and a straightforward incision of the space is well justified.

In controlled situations when the skin has been infiltrated with local anaesthetic, an incision is made in the skin-marked area and the opening is widened with scissors. Blunt tissue separation with an artery forceps or McIndoe scissors will reveal the cricothyroid membrane. As soon as the cricothyroid membrane is found it is incised in the line of the skin incision and the area is dilated with an artery forceps or with a tracheostomy dilator (Fig. 29.2).

It is essential to avoid injuries to the cartilages. The average cricothyroidostomy aperture can easily accommodate a No. 6 tracheostomy tube. Once the tube has been positioned properly, the skin is allowed to fall back on it. Skin should not be sutured on the sides of the tracheostomy tube. Such skin closure will usually result in subcutaneous emphysema and related problems.

The space is very limited and if prolonged intubation is maintained through this cricothyroidostomy then subglottic stenosis may result. Therefore if intubation is required for longer than 48 hours then within 48 hours, the cricothyroidostomy should be replaced with a formal tracheostomy.

The care of the cricothyroidostomy is the same as that of a tracheostomy (see section 30).

30 Tracheostomy

If an injury to the larynx is suspected, and if the condition of the patient is such that prolonged intubation is deemed necessary, then a tracheostomy should be performed at the outset. Formal tracheostomy takes much longer than cricothyroidostomy and if life is in jeopardy then cricothyroidostomy is to be preferred. If, however, the patient's condition is stabilised, then tracheostomy is much more reliable and is much more easy to manage.

If spinal cord injury has not been excluded then neck movement such as flexion and extension should be avoided during X-rays and tracheostomy (see section 26).

The protocol of performing a tracheostomy is the same as that of cricothyroidostomy. The patient's neck is prepared antiseptically with povidone iodine or with chlorhexidine solution in alcohol. After towelling, draping and isolating the proposed site of tracheostomy, a skin incision is marked with indelible ink.

The preferred approach for tracheostomy is via a transverse 3 cm long incision placed midway between the cricoid cartilage and the suprasternal notch (Fig. 30.1).

With patients in whom sternomastoid cannot be palpated due to haematoma or laceration, and in whom other landmarks are also not easily found, a vertical incision is preferable. The skin is infiltrated with adrenaline/lignocaine solution (1:100,000, 1% lignocaine 5 ml). After raising a wheal the skin is horizontally incised for 3 cm until the edges of the sternomastoid are found. Lignocaine 0.5% without adrenaline, is then infiltrated into the depths of the wound. The sternomastoid on either side are retracted away. The middle cervical fascia is

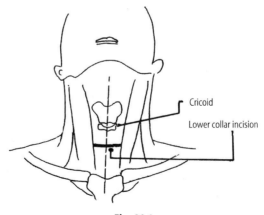

Cricoid

Lower collar incision

Fig. 30.1

117

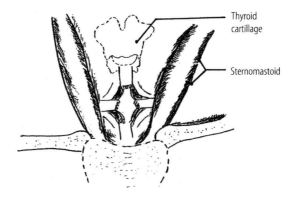

Wide resection for tracheostomy

Fig. 30.2

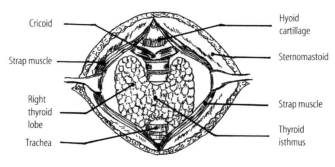

Fig. 30.3

incised vertically. The incised margins of the middle cervical fascia with the medial margins of sternohyoid muscle are retracted away laterally. The exposed area is then deepened and cleared by blunt dissection with an artery forceps (Fig. 30.2). Following this separation, the thyroid isthmus is dissected posteriorly and through large artery forceps, the isthmus is clamped on either side and divided in the middle (Fig. 30.3). With midline division of the

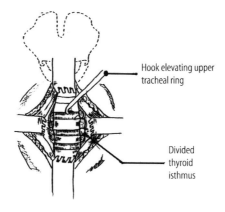

Fig. 30.4

isthmus, the clamped area of the isthmus is then ligated haemostatically using continuous chromic catgut or Vicaryl 2/0. Once the isthmus is haemostatically ligated, then it is retracted on either side to reveal the second and the third tracheal rings/cartilages (Fig. 30.4).

The ideal area to perform the tracheostomy is between the second and the third rings of the trachea. In order to stabilise the trachea and to prevent its movement while midline incisions are being made, a skin hook is used to fix the lower border of the first tracheal cartilage. This maintains the trachea in one position and with this tracheal hook in position, self-retaining retractors are now applied separating away the thyroid isthmus and the adjacent muscles (Fig. 30.5).

Subsequent tracheal stenosis can be avoided and good healing ensured by raising a flap of trachea through which the tracheostomy tube can be inserted. This is performed by horizontally incising the trachea between the first and the second tracheal rings. Similar horizontal incision is made in the space between the third and the fourth tracheal rings.

A vertical incision is next made across the tracheal cartilages joining the horizontal incisions in the midline and cutting through the second and the third tracheal cartilages. A good fine sucker must be kept alongside to aspirate any bleeding. As soon as the trachea is opened, the respiratory pattern changes. Mucus secretions and any bleeding should be aspirated quickly.

A tracheostomy dilator or separator is inserted, moving the flaps on either side and through this the tracheostomy tube can be inserted. Before the tracheostomy tube is inserted, it is a good policy to fix the tracheal flap with strong Prolene stay sutures (size 0) on either side and then to leave these untied and long, attached with a skin tape. This is very useful in cases where the tracheostomy tube falls out accidentally. With traction of the Prolene sutures tied to the tracheal flap on either side, the tracheostomy aperture becomes easily accessible for reinsertion of the tracheal tube.

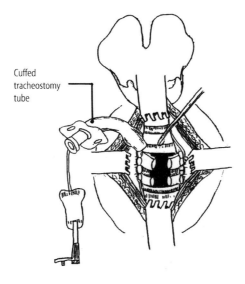

Cuffed tracheostomy tube

Divided tracheal ring

Fig. 30.5

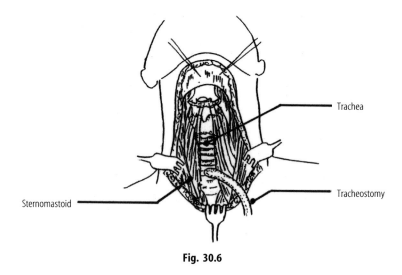

Fig. 30.6

An appropriate-sized tracheostomy tube is inserted and the plastic flanges of the tube are stitched to the sides of the skin wound. In order to prevent subcutaneous emphysema, the skin incision should not be closed around the tracheostomy tightly. A circumferential cervical tape is looped around the back of the neck and is anchored to the tracheostomy flange on either side (Fig. 30.6).

Sterile suction catheters are introduced to aspirate any blood or sputum from the lower end of the trachea. The tracheostomy tube cuff is then inflated with air to prevent aspiration of saliva.

Intermittently, the trachea should be cleared with a disposable sterile sucker. The tube should be kept meticulously clean and covered with a porous sterile gauze. When the patient is unconscious, humidified oxygen is supplied via a sterile tube. In an alert patient, the humidification should be provided by moistening of the gauze or by providing steam nearby. The aspirate or the sputum should be periodically cultured. Chest physiotherapy should be provided regularly. If an endotracheal cuff has been inflated then this should be periodically deflated to prevent tracheal necrosis but just prior to this, a thorough aspiration must be done to prevent inhalation of retained mucus.

When the need of a tracheostomy ends, the tracheostomy should be intermittently plugged with an obturator. If normal breathing is possible then the tracheostomy tube is removed and the orifice covered with sterile gauze. The withdrawn tracheal flap of cartilage falls back into place and within a few days time no tracheal leak is apparent!

Tracheal stenosis is a common problem following a prolonged tracheostomy. This is largely unpreventable unless tracheal flaps are routinely raised, as described above.

Percutaneous tracheostomy using large bore needles can also be used in emergencies. Using dilators, the aperture can be enlarged until a fair-sized tube can be inserted.

31 Laryngeal Injuries

The larynx comprises the following cartilages which are bonded together as a single integral functional unit:

- thyroid cartilage
- cricoid cartilage
- epiglottis
- arytenoid cartilage (paired)
- cuneiform cartilage
- corniculate cartilage.

The thyroid cartilage, whose upper border lies at the level of the adult fifth cervical vertebra, is the largest component of the larynx, consisting of two large laminae joined anteriorily at an acute angle. This junction protrudes as a prominence (Adam's apple). The projection of this angle varies with age and sex. The angle is greater in females (110–120°) and lesser in the males (90°). Above the prominence, the V-shaped thyroid notch separates the laminae. The posterior parts of the laminae radiate out into two projections or processes called the superior and the inferior horns. The superior horn turns backwards and medially to end as a cone into which the lateral thyrohyoid ligament is attached. This ligament often contains a triticeous cartilage. The inferior horn is much shorter and broader and at its lower end contains an oval facet for articulation with the side of the cricoid cartilage.

The cricoid cartilage is thicker, much smaller but stronger in substance than the thyroid cartilage. It is the only firm structure that fully encircles the respiratory passage. The anterior part of the cartilage is narrow and the posterior part is broader and forms the quadrate lamina.

The arytenoid cartilage is a paired structure and articulates with the upper border of the quadrate lamina of the cricoid cartilage. The arytenoid cartilage narrows anteriorly into a pyramidal process. An anterior projecting part of this pyramidal process is called the vocal process that is connected to the vocal fold. A laterally projecting part of the pyramidal process is called the muscular process into which are attached the posterior and the lateral crico-arytenoid muscles. The upper border of the arytenoid cartilage articulates with the corniculate cartilage which gives attachment to the aryepiglottic fold. This fold contains the cuneiform cartilage.

The epiglottis is a thin fibroelastic cartilaginous projection behind the tongue and the body of the hyoid bone. It is attached below to the thyroepiglottic ligament. The sides of the epiglottis are attached by the aryepiglottic folds to the arytenoid cartilage. The epiglottis is covered by mucous membrane.

The most common type of blunt laryngeal injury seen nowadays is caused by road traffic accidents (RTAs). However, when other injuries to the body are adjusted with such statistics, the incidence of isolated laryngeal injuries with RTAs is very small. Most such RTA laryngeal injuries are complicated with injuries to additional structures (chest, skull, limbs or face). Many RTA injuries to the anterior aspect of the neck are instantly fatal. Despite the use of a helmet, motorcycle falls often produce closed injuries to the larynx.[71]

Another common non-criminal mechanism of laryngeal injury is a blunt trauma to the anterior surface of the neck, caused by an accidental fall from a height.

Iatrogenic laryngeal injury may occur with endotracheal intubation, laryngoscopy, endoscopy, local neck surgery, tracheostomy, cricothyroidostomy and so on.

Criminal violence (bullet injury, shotgun injuries, clubbing, kicking while the victim is on the ground, attempted strangulation, stabs) or suicide attempts with a knife are common criminal causes of laryngeal injuries.

After a trauma to the neck the suspicion of a laryngeal injury arises from certain suspect symptoms such as dysphonia, aphonia, dyspnoea, stridor, haemoptysis, pain in the neck, dysphagia, or odynophagia.

On clinical examination, there may be a swelling present in the neck or there may be a change present in the contour of the neck, with loss of anatomical landmarks. There may be tenderness present with crepitus. Subcutaneous emphysema may be visible or palpable.

The main life-threatening problems of such an injury are asphyxia, haemorrhage and spinal cord injury.

Patients presenting with manifest laryngeal injuries should be suspected for vertebral or spinal cord injuries and these should be excluded by a thorough neurological examination and appropriate X-rays or scans of the cervical spine. If the condition of the patient is such that emergency cricothyroidostomy or tracheostomy is necessary prior to radiological exclusion of vertebral injuries then this must be so performed as to avoid aggravation of an associated cervical vertebral injury. Neck flexion should be avoided.

When an emergency cricothyroidostomy has been performed, it should be converted (within 48 hours) to a tracheostomy, when the condition of the patient is stabilised and it is deemed that airway management should be thus maintained for a prolonged period of time.

If laryngeal injuries are clinically suspected then instead of an endotracheal intubation or a cricothyroidostomy, a tracheostomy is preferable. This will keep the airway a safe distance away from the site of the injury.

If vertebral injury has been excluded and there is no contraindication to neck flexion and extension, then with a suspicion of laryngeal injuries the endolarynx should be assessed by laryngoscopy. This can be easily performed and if there is any evidence of a significant laryngeal damage present, then a tracheostomy should be performed forthwith.

If facilities exist, then computerised tomography (CT) scans of the larynx are also helpful. If the condition of the patient is compromised in respect of the airway, then a tracheostomy must be performed immediately and assessment of the cervical spinal cord and endolarynx must be done subsequently.

If there are features present of laryngeal structural deformities etc, then a proper exploration and repair of the damaged area is necessary as soon as the patient's general condition and respiration have improved. The best way of administering anaesthesia is via a tracheostomy performed either under a local or general anaesthetic. Mask anaesthesia is given with airway protection for a brief period and rapid tracheostomy is established. Translaryngeal intubation is dangerous and may exacerbate the injury. Once tracheostomy anaesthesia has commenced and the patient is adequately draped, surgery can begin. For planned operations on the larynx, a high transverse curving incision (see XX in Fig. 31.1) is best. Via this incision, tissue damage is minimal and exposure of laryngeal skeleton and endolarynx is rapid.

The disadvantage of this high collar incision is that other structures such as trachea and oesophagus cannot be adequately exposed. With the planned incision for laryngeal exposure (XX), the upper flap is elevated to the hyoid cartilage. The hyoid cartilage is examined next. It is palpated for fractures and if palpation is unreliable (haematoma, bruising) then the perichondrium overlying the hyoid cartilage is incised with a sharp-pointed knife. The perichondrium is then elevated using a Freer perichondrial elevator. The intrinsic muscular attachment is also freed. When a fracture is found its full extent is assessed and any loose and devascularised pieces removed. The fracture is wired using a fine (30-gauge) interosseous wire (Fig. 31.2).

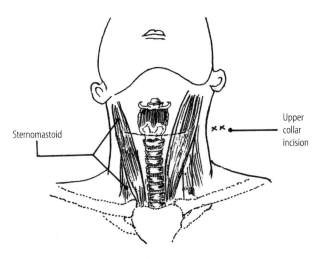

Fig. 31.1

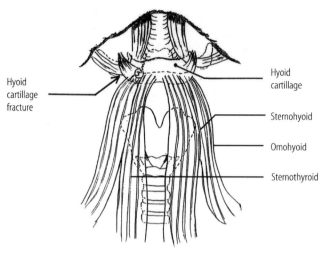

Hyoid cartillage fracture

Hyoid cartillage

Sternohyoid

Omohyoid

Sternothyroid

Fig. 31.2

The thyroid cartilage is inspected next. Once the strap muscles have been retracted, the perichondrium of the thyroid cartilage is vertically incised with a sharp knife. Using Freer's perichondrial elevator, the thyroid perichondrium is elevated on either side from the thyroid notch down to the cricothyroid membrane. The cricothyroid membrane is preserved. The perichondrium overlying the cricoid cartilage is similarly elevated to the sides. Usually brisk bleeding may result from ruptured cricothyroid arteries on either side and bipolar cautery controls it easily. Once thyroid fractures are encountered, it is a good policy to inspect the endolarynx to check for internal injuries. If facilities for peroperative endoscopic endolaryngeal examination are available then open exposure of the larynx can be avoided. If endoscopic evidence exists for mucosal damage requiring sutures or if endoscopy is not available then thyrotomy must be done to directly inspect the interior and to undertake immediate repair.

Using a Stryker or a dental saw, the midline part of perichondrium-denuded thyroid cartilage is cut cleanly down to the cricothyroid membrane. The thyrotomy must be performed gently and the underlying mucosa should not be damaged (Fig. 31.3).

At this stage the cricothyroid membrane is incised with a fine-pointed scalpel (size 15 blade) vertically. Using cartilage hooks on either side, the thyroid cartilage is retracted to expose the endolarynx. If mucosal tear is found then this is repaired using 5/0 or 6/0 catgut. If mucosal loss is substantial, then a mucosal graft should be used to close the defects (Fig. 31.4).

Once the endolaryngeal mucosa has been repaired, the dislocated arytenoid cartilages should be replaced and stabilised with fine wires. If the epiglottis is found injured, it can be repaired or sutured to the base of the tongue. If it cannot be repaired easily then it should be amputated and the defect closed with absorbable sutures (Fig. 31.5).

Once the mucosa of the endolarynx has been repaired all around, the retracted thyroid and cricoid cartilages are brought close together. Fractures and midline thyrotomy can be easily

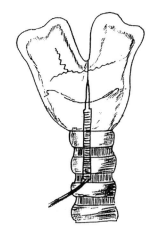

Thyroitomy saw

Fig. 31.3

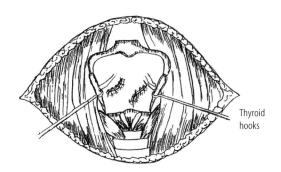

Thyroid
hooks

Mucosal tear repaired

Fig. 31.4

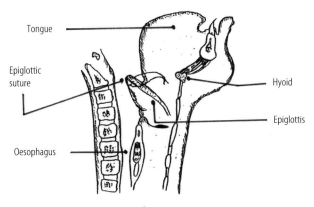

Tongue

Epiglottic
suture

Hyoid

Epiglottis

Oesophagus

Fig. 31.5

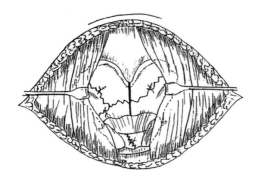

Fracture of thyroid cartillage

Fig. 31.6

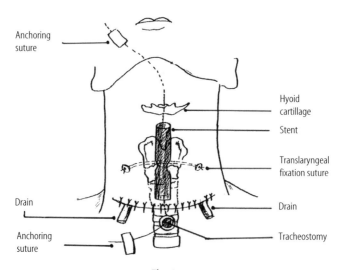

Anchoring suture

Hyoid cartillage

Stent

Translaryngeal fixation suture

Drain

Drain

Anchoring suture

Tracheostomy

Fig. 31.7

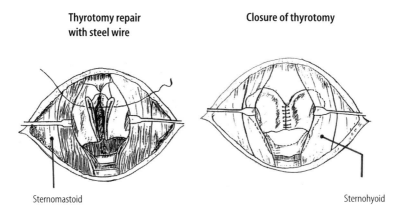

Thyrotomy repair with steel wire

Closure of thyrotomy

Sternomastoid

Sternohyoid

Fig. 31.8

reduced and reapproximated using fine wire. It is important to repair the cartilages extramucosally and therefore repair should be done under vision. A good technique is to insert wires and to leave them untied to the last. In a young patient, the steel wire needles can perforate the margins of the thyroid and cricoid cartilages, but when these cartilages are more "osseous" then holes must be drilled using a fine dental burr. The mucosa must not be perforated. If it is accidentally perforated then it should be repaired at once otherwise a fistula may result. Once all of the wires (No. 30 stainless steel wire) have been applied, these are properly and systematically tied, ensuring that fracture reductions remain secure and stable (Fig. 31.6).

A laryngeal stent should be inserted to prevent stenosis. Prefabricated stents are ideal but a stent can be easily improvised using a silastic endotracheal tube. The upper lumen is closed off using strong Prolene. A central anchoring suture of Prolene is brought out through the mouth and is firmly secured to skin. The lower end is similarly tied off and another central Prolene suture is exteriorised through the tracheostomy orifice.

The aim of the stent-implantation is to prevent stenosis and therefore it must be implanted in the correct position. It should extend both above and below the laryngeal fracture, but should not extend to the tracheostomy orifice. It should fit loosely at the greatest laryngeal constriction. At this point a large Prolene suture is passed percutaneously from one side of the neck, going across skin, muscles, larynx, stent and coming out through stent, larynx, muscles and skin of the opposite side. Both ends of this Prolene suture are anchored to skin using crushed beads and buttons. The stent is thus secured above, below and transversely (Fig. 31.7).

The perichondrium is closed over thyroid and cricoid cartilages. Cricothyroid membrane is securely repaired. Strap muscles are allowed to fall back on their respective sides. Drains (vacuum) are exteriorised from the deep plane on either side to the side of the neck and securely anchored to skin with Prolene or silk sutures. Drains should be removed, if no significant bleeding results after 24 hours, to prevent exogenous infection (Fig. 31.8).

32 Tracheal Injuries

A complete rupture of the cervical trachea can occur without an external neck injury being visible.[72] Usually an anteroposterior directed mechanical force (road traffic accident (RTA), assault, and so on) compresses the trachea against the cervical spine[73] disrupting it, usually at one level but rupture of the trachea can also occur during straining at labour or during a bout of coughing to dislodge a foreign body.[74]

Even a small tracheal rupture can lead to severe complications and therefore if airway has become compromised then surgical intervention becomes essential. In only a few rare cases, when the extent of the tracheal damage is minimal, does a simple conservative follow-up observation become justified. Common clinical features of tracheal injuries include stridor, haemoptysis and subcutaneous air-emphysema.

Most tracheal injuries are potentially curable and the delay in offering treatment results in increased morbidity (aspiration and infection) and mortality. Both can be averted with timely intervention.

Once again, it must be emphasised that isolated tracheal injury is rare and usually an injury forceful enough to cause tracheal damage is nearly always associated with other injuries such as to thyroid, larynx, oesophagus and to the neurovascular structures in the neck.

Tracheal injury

Direct repair of trachea
with in-situ orotracheal tube

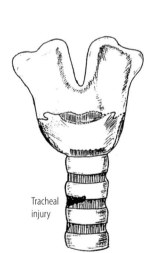

Tracheal injury

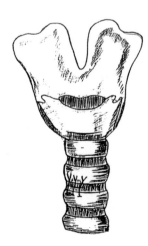

Fig. 32.1

If the diagnosis is pure tracheal injury (caused mainly by knife stabs and so on) then a cervical collar incision is adequate under a formal general anaesthesia delivered either via a tracheostomy or through an orotracheal tube. The thyroid isthmus is divided as described above and the upper tracheal rings exposed. Dissection is carried down to the lowest possible level. If the tracheal leak is not easily visible then saline is poured over the wound cavity and the patient is ventilated by bag after deflating the endotracheal tube cuff. This allows air to bubble through and the puncture is easily identified. All necrotic or ischaemic tissue is removed and then repair is undertaken using Dexon or Vicaryl sutures (2/0 or 3/0). If an entire ring of trachea is devitalised then this is dissected clean.

The blood supply of the trachea mainly enters from the sides (principally from the inferior thyroid artery) and bilateral sharp dissections should be avoided, if possible.

Membranous tracheal sutures are first taken and held by artery forceps. Cartilaginous bites are taken next and these are also held with artery forceps (Fig. 32.1).

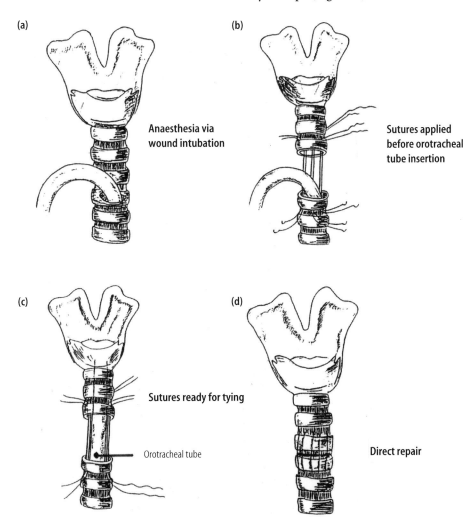

Fig. 32.2

With the orotracheal tube in position (placed caudal to the tracheal damage), all of the sutures are tied and the anastomosis rechecked with saline and air as described earlier. If the available space allows it, a decompression tracheostomy is created caudal to the tracheal repair but this is not essential. If decompression tracheostomy has not been performed then postoperatively endotracheal or orotracheal tube is removed soon. Tracheal repairs heal very quickly but antibiotic cover must be provided for prophylaxis against infections. If the tracheal ring is non-viable and necrosis in the adjoining area intense, then the entire ring needs to be excised with restoration of air passage.

An endotracheal tube is quickly inserted through the wound into the trachea and anaesthesia commenced (Fig. 32.2a). The necrotic trachea is quickly excised and appropriate sutures passed through from above and below the cartilages for security (Fig. 32.2b). An orotracheal tube is then negotiated past the damaged area and the previous tube removed (Fig. 32.2c). Sutures are now tied and intervening sutures are applied to securely close the defects (Fig. 32.2d).

33 Injuries to the Cervical Oesophagus

External injuries to the oesophagus from penetrating trauma are rare. Of the overall injuries to the oesophagus approximately 60% occur in the cervical portion and many of these are associated with concomitant injuries to the regional structures such as the trachea, larynx, the great vessels and the regional nerves.[75]

The commonest reported oesophageal injuries are from diagnostic or therapeutic instrumentation. Haematoma, partial laceration or perforation can occur with any form of instrumentation. Surprisingly, some of the most severe form of injuries are seen with difficult endotracheal intubation and with the forced passage of nasogastric tubes. In a large study, 72% perforations occurred from various iatrogenic causes, of which 60% were in the cervical oesophagus, 30% were in the mid-thoracic and only 1% was in the distal oesophagus.[76]

Cervical oesophageal perforations secondary to instrumentations are located principally over the cricopharyngeus muscle on the posterior wall. Here the oesophagus is thin walled owing to absence of longitudinal muscle fibres and has marked narrowing of the lumen at the introitus. Repeated hyperextension of the neck, kyphosis or spondylitic osteophytes may exaggerate the pressure of oesophagus against the cervical vertebra and may predispose to injury at this level.[76]

Therapeutic oesophageal dilatations for strictures can result in perforation. The highest incidence of such iatrogenic perforations is recorded with pneumatic dilators, followed closely by those caused with metal olives and lowest with mercury-weighted bougies. Bad anaesthesia, bad technique and poor preparation are contributing causes of oesophageal injury.[17]

Penetrating knife and glass injuries are rare modes of injury. Bullet injuries can also cause oesophageal perforation.

In the usual course of events, oesophageal injuries are occult on initial presentation and frank mediastinitis and local sepsis become manifest much later. Dysphagia, odynophagia or a swelling which occurs on swallowing fluids are features of oesophageal perforation.

Since mediastinal pressure is subatmospheric during normal breathing, a tear of oesophagus can lead to suction of luminal contents directly into the potential mediastinal space. This perioesophageal space is readily infected because the tissue is poorly vascularised. Anaerobic organisms proliferate quickly. Mediastinitis can range from diffuse cellulitis to frank suppuration. This infection can extend from the cranial vault to the diaphragm.

Since the morbidity and mortality of oesophageal perforation are very high, it is imperative to exercise an aggressive policy. If platysma has been severed and any of the clinical features of oesophageal injuries are seen, the area must be explored to exclude an oesophageal injury. Gastrografin swallow, dye tests and so on are unreliable in many such injuries.

Even if an exploration for suspected oesophageal perforation has eventually been found to be negative, the operative trauma is well worth inflicting because the dangers from an untreated oesophageal tear far outweigh the small risks of negative surgical exploration in the right hands. The best access to a suspected or a confirmed oesophageal injury is via an oblique cervical incision (Fig. 33.1).

The sternomastoid is retracted laterally. The inferolateral lobe of thyroid is retracted medially and in the process, the inferior thyroid artery is ligated. The carotid sheath is displaced inferiorly and laterally. The omohyoid is divided. This allows a good access to the cervical oesophagus. The cricopharyngeus muscle and recurrent laryngeal nerve should be preserved (the left nerve commonly being in the groove between the oesophagus and trachea and the right one being on the anterolateral surface of the upper cervical oesophagus) (Fig. 33.2).

Repair of minor tears can be undertaken using Lembert non-absorbable sutures (3/0 silk) in one layer (Fig. 33.3).

Larger tears or complete division of oesophagus should be surgically treated formally with a two-layer closure after debridement and freshening of the margins. The inner layer is closed with 3/0 Dexon or Vicaryl. The outer layer is closed with alternating interrupted horizontal mattress and Lembert sutures of 3/0 silk (Fig. 33.4).

If both trachea and oesophagus are injured at the same level, then through this incision, both these viscera can be adequately repaired. In such an eventuality, the distal trachea should be

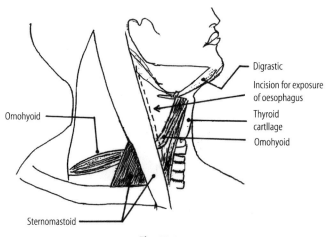

Fig. 33.1

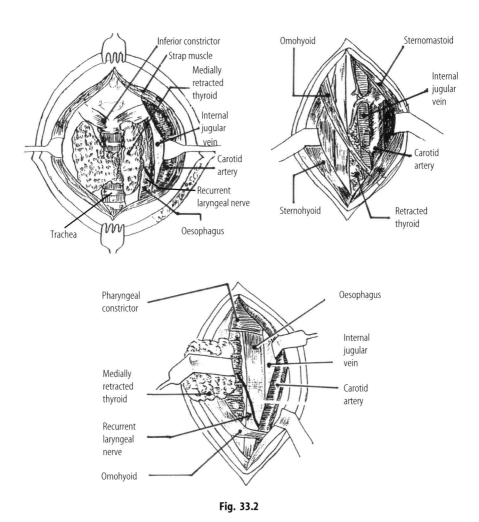

Fig. 33.2

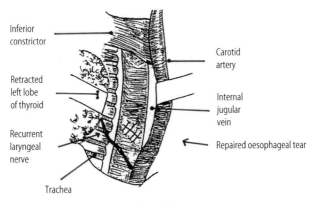

Fig. 33.3

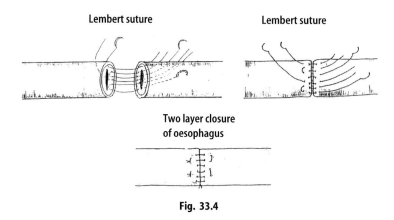

Fig. 33.4

decompressed with a tracheostomy and the oesophageal repair should be protected with a decompressing nasogastric tube. Into the intervening area between these two repairs a vascularised flap of sternomastoid or sternohyoid muscle should be inserted (Fig. 33.5). A fistula is thus prevented between the viscera. The repaired area must be drained liberally, if necessary with two drains which should be removed if there is no substantial bleeding or leakage seen after 24 hours.

With such oesophageal injuries, parenteral antibiotics (a combination of cephalosporin/ metronidazole and penicillin) and parenteral nutrition, for a week should continue, although the nasogastric tube may be removed on the second or the third day.

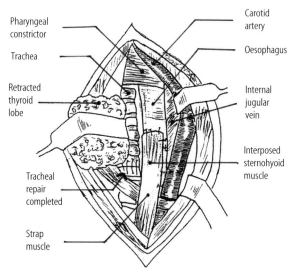

Fig. 33.5

34 References

1 Smith E. *Papyrus*. Birmingham, AL: Classics of Surgery Library, 1984.

2 Robbs JV, Keenan J. Exploration of the neck: operative surgery. *Robbs' and Smith's trauma surgery*, 4th edn. London: Butterworths, 1989, p 106.

3 Trunkey DD. *Trauma principles and penetrating neck trauma: Current therapy of trauma*. Trunkey, Lewis eds. London: Mosby, 1984, pp 79–83.

4 Schultz RC. Mechanisms, characterization and incidence of injuries. In: *Facial injuries*, 2nd edn. Chicago, IL: Year Book Medical Publishers, 1977, pp 12–14.

5 Vincent JM, Di Maio. In *Gunshot wounds*. New York: Elsevier, 1985, pp 1–32.

6 Levin LJ. In: *Ballistics of bullet injury: Operative surgery: Trauma surgery*, 4th edn. London: Butterworths, 1989, pp 106–110.

7 Coates JB , Beyer JC. *Wound ballistics, Medical Department of the US Army in WWI*. Washington, DC: Office of the Surgeon General of the Department of the Army, 1962.

8 McSwain NE. *Penetrating Neck Wounds. Major advances in the 1980s*. Chicago, IL: Year Book Medical Publishers, 1986, pp 135–156.

9 Baker S *et al*. *The injury fact book*. Lexington, 1984, pp 219–251.

10 Trunkey DD. Current therapy of trauma. 1984–85. *General approach to the injured patient*. London: Mosby.

11 Fischer H, Kirkpatrick CJ. *A colour atlas of trauma pathology*. London: Wolfe Publishing, 1991, pp 31–71.

12 Rich NM. Vascular trauma. *Surg Clin N Am* **53**: 1367–92, 1973.

13 Patrick LM. Studies of hyperextension and hyperflexion injury in volunteers and human cadavers. *Neckache and backache*. Springfield, IL, 1970, pp 92–107.

14 Larson SJ. In extensive acceleration injuries. In *Neurological surgery*, Vol 4. 3rd edn. Youmans JR ed. WB Saunders, 1990, pp 2392–2402.

15 Mackay M. Kinematics of vehicle crashes. In *Advances in trauma*, Vol 2. Maulk I *et al*. eds. Chicago, IL: Year Book Medical Publishers, 1987, pp 21–42.

16 Hollinger PH *et al*. Internal and external trauma to larynx. *Laryngoscope* **78**: 944–954, 1968.

17 Vanezis P. Toxic and miscellaneous environmental causes of neck injuries. In *Pathology of neck injuries*. London: Butterworths, 1989.

18 Suechting R, French LA. PICA syndrome following fracture of cervical vertebra. *J Neurosurg* **12**: 187–189, 1955.

19 Zimmerman AW, Kumar AJ, Gadoth V *et al.* Traumatic vertebrobasilar occlusive disease in childhood. *Neurology* **28**: 185–188, 1978.

20 Babar SMA. Traumatic extracranial vertebral artery aneurysm. A case report and review of literature. *Pak Heart J* **19**(4): 75–82, 1986.

21 Krueger BR, Okazaki H. Vertebral-basilar distribution infarction following chiropractic cervical manipulation. *Mayo Clin Proc* **55**: 322–332, 1980.

22 Babar SMA. Aneurysms of the upper limb. *Ind Pract* **44**(12): 949–958, 1991.

23 Silverman *et al.* The dynamics of transient cerebral blindness. Report of nine episodes. *Arch Neurologica* **4**: 330–348, 1961.

24 Sugar O *et al.* Vertebral angiography. *Am J Roentgen* **61**: 166–182, 1949.

25 Morgan RNW, Morrel DF. Internal jugular catheterisation. *Anaesthesia* **36**: 512–517, 1981.

26 Gamulin Z, Bruckner JC, Forster A *et al.* Multiple complications after internal jugular vein catheterisation. *Anaesthesia* **41**: 408–412, 1986.

27 Stell PM, Morrison MD. Radiation necrosis of the larynx. Etiology and management. *Arch Otolaryng* **98**: 11–113, 1973.

28 Mills M. Early treatment of spinal injuries. In *A colour atlas of accident and emergencies.* Weert: Wolfe, 1984.

29 Committee on Trauma. Early care of the injured patient, "Neck" chapter. *A.C. Surg.* 2nd edn. WB Saunders, 1976, pp 149–160.

30 Feliciano DV, Bitondo OG, Mattox KL *et al.* Civilian trauma in the 1980s. A 10 year experience with 456 vascular and cardiac injuries. *Ann Surg* **199**: 717–724, 1984.

31 Merger D *et al.* Vertebral artery trauma. Acute recognition and treatment. *Arch Surg* **116**: 236–239, 1981.

32 Feliciano DV. Vascular injuries. *Advances in trauma 2.* Chicago, IL: Year Book Medical Publishers, 1987, pp 179–206.

33 Brown MF, Graham JH, Feliciano DV *et al.* Carotid artery injuries. *Am J Surg* **144**: 748–753, 1982.

34 Beatty RA. Dissecting haematoma of the ICA following chiropractic cervical manipulation. *J Trauma* **17**: 248–249, 1977.

35 Babar SMA, Ansari AA, Ramadan SA. How should we investigate TIA? *Cent African J Med* **37**(3): 90–103, 1991.

36 Najafi H, Javid H, Dye WS *et al.* Emergency carotid thromboendarterectomy. *Arch Surg* **106**: 520, 1973.

37 Hunter JA *et al.* Emergency operations for acute cerebral ischaemia due to carotid artery obstruction. Review of 26 cases. *Ann Surg* **162**: 901, 1965.

38 Rob CJ, Wheeler EB. Thrombosis of ICA treated by arterial surgery. *Br Med J* **2**: 264, 1957.

39 Haimovici H. Vascular emergencies. In *Haemorhagic and thrombotic disorders.* Appleton-Century Crofts, 1982, pp 65–85.

40 Goldstein P. Fatal interstitial and mediastinal emphysema. *Am J Dis Children* **78**: 375–383, 1949.

41 Babar SMA. Peripheral pseudoaneurysms in a third world country. *J Vasc Surg* **27**(4): 253–263, 1993.

42 Miller DC, Roon AJ. Diagnosis and management of peripheral vascular disease. In *Aneurysms*. Addison-Wesley 1982, pp 199–210.

43 Babar SMA. One-stage reconstruction of peripheral neurovascular gunshot injuries in a third world country. *J Vasc Surg* **28**(1): 29–38, 1994.

44 Babar SMA. Carotid paraganglioma. *Pak J Cardiology* **3**: 23–30, 1991.

45 Bell PRF, Barrie W. *Operative arterial surgery*. Bristol: Wright, 1981, pp 56–57.

46 Babar SMA. Peripheral neurovascular injuries. *Ind Pract* **45**(9): 725–741, 1992.

47 Doniach I, Williams ED. Biological effects of radiation on the thyroid. In *Thyroid*, 5th edn. Ingbarr SH, Braverman LE eds. Philadelphia, PA: Lippincott, 1986, Chapter 17.

48 Vanezis P. *Pathology of neck injury*. London: Butterworths, 1989. Chapter 13.

49 Saternus KS. The mechanism of whiplash injury of the cervical spine. *Zentralblatt Rechtsmmedizin* **88**: 1–11, 1982.

50 Hucklestep PR. *A simple guide to trauma*, 4th edn. Churchill Livingstone, 1986, pp 253–262.

51 Dolan EJ, Tator CH, Endrenyi L *et al*. The value of decompression for acute experimental spinal cord compression injury. *J Neurosurg* **53**: 749–764, 1980.

52 Carter and Polk. Craniocervical injury. In *Surgery 1 (Trauma)*. Butterworths, London, 1981, pp 40–65.

53 Templeton and Wilson. In *Lecture notes on trauma*. Oxford: Blackwell Scientific, 1983, pp 17–19.

54 Kajihara K, Kawanaga H, De la Torre JC *et al*. DMSO in the treatment of experimental acute spinal cord injury. *Surg Neurologica* **1**: 16, 1973.

55 Panganamala RV, Sharma HM, Heikkila RE *et al*. Role of hydroxyl radical scavengers, DMSO, alcohol and methional in the inhibition of prostaglandin biosynthesis. *Prostaglandin* **11**: 599, 1976.

56 Kao C *et al*. Axonal regeneration across transected mammalian spinal cords. An EM study of delayed microsurgical nerve grafting. *Exp Neurologica* **54**: 591, 1977.

57 Richardson P *et al*. Peripheral nerve autografts to the rat spinal cord. Studies with axon tracing methods. *Brain Res* **237**: 147, 1982.

58 Hallas B. Transplantation into the mammalian adult spinal cord. *Experimentia* **38**: 699, 1982.

59 Babar SMA. One-stage repair of subclavian pseudoaneurysm and brachial plexus injury. *Med Pract Dec* 7–20, 1990.

60 Sunderland S. *Nerves and nerve injuries*, 2nd edn. Churchill Livingstone, 1978.

61 Brown HA. The value of early neurolysis in contused injuries of peripheral nerves. *Western J Surg* **61**: 535–37, 1953.

62 Sakellorides H. Follow-up of 172 peripheral nerve injuries in upper extremity in civilians. *J Bone Joint Surg* **44A**: 140–148, 1962.

63 Kline DG, Hudson AR. Acute injuries of the peripheral nerves. In *Neurological surgery*. Vol 4, 3rd edn. London: WB Saunders, 1990.

64 Kline DG, Hackett E. Reappraisal of timing for exploration of civilian peripheral nerve injuries. *Surgery* **78**: 54–65, 1975.

65 Babar SMA. Axillary aneurysm and brachial plexus lesion. *Pak J Med Res* **30**(1): 46–58, 1991.

66 Millesi H. Brachial plexus injuries: Nerve grafting. *Clin Orthop* **237**: 36–42, 1988.

67 Merrem G, Goldhahn WE. *Surgery of peripheral nervous system*. In *Neurosurgical operations*, Goldhahn WE ed. Translated by Telger TC. Springer-Verlag, 1981.

68 Merrem G. *Neurosurgical operations*, 2nd edn. Springer-Verlag, 1981.

69 Yarlington CT. Trauma involving the air and food passages. *Otolaryng Clin N Am* **12**: 251–469, 1979.

70 Edgerton MT Jr. Emergency care of maxillofacial and neck injuries. In *The management of trauma*. London: WB Saunders, 1973, pp 255–321.

71 Angood PB, Attia EL, Brown RA *et al*. Extrinsic civilian trauma to the larynx and cervical trachea. Important predictors of long term morbidity. *J Trauma* **26**: 869–873, 1986.

72 Coetzee T *et al*. Complete subcutaneous rupture-separation of cervical trachea. *J Trauma* **5**: 458–463, 1965.

73 Arora YR. Closed cervical tracheal rupture. *Br J Clin Pract* **17**: 341–342, 1963.

74 Zench LH. Subcutaneous rupture of the trachea. *Illin Med J* **41**: 451–454.

75 Carter D, Polk H. *Surgery (Trauma)*. London: Butterworths, 1981, pp 78–82.

76 Norman EA, Sosis M. Iatrogenic oesophageal perforation due to tracheal or nasogastric intubation. *Can Anaesth Soc J* **33**: 222–226, 1986.

Index